No Drama

-

TODDLER SLEEP TRAINING

Gently way to train toddler for a healthy sleep.

By Ann M. Watson

TABLE OF CONTENTS

INTRODUCTION

At all ages, sleep, in enough quantity and quality, helps recover from the physical and nervous fatigue of the day. In children, it is beneficial for their development, growth, the functioning of the immune system, and the establishment of nervous circuits, memorization, and learning.

Nowadays, with the invention of streetlights on the roads, society has appropriated being awake at night, and the rhythm of sleep is not the same as before. Also, the technological palette (smartphone, tablet, computer, etc.) tends to disrupt our sleep cycles more and more. Generally, the internal clock is regulated by the alternation of the day and the night. All electronic devices carrying artificial light sends false messages to our brains.

Also, stress has a significant impact on an individual's sleep. Since today's society involves a lot of movement, whether at work or in private life, this can cause stress for parents. People must manage their private life as well as work while being concerned with the busy schedule of their children. The latter being emotional "sponges," they feel the tensions or the anxieties of those around them. So that the child can have a restful sleep, it is preferable that he grow up in a favorable environment and that he feels safe.

The child does not sleep on command or because we put him to bed. It is essential to watch for signals that may signal the need for sleep. Be aware that each child has individual signs. Also, sleep time varies according to the different needs of the children of their age.

CHAPTER ONE

Introduction to Development.

For the realization of this point, we decided to start with a small introduction to sleep. We chose to organize the book according to the age group of the child. The first part will be dedicated to babies, from birth to eighteen months, and the second part will be devoted to children aged eighteen months to three years.

Sleep.

The duration of sleep, the manner of sleeping, and the cycles are specific to each. All of this evolves throughout life. Many studies have been done since the 1960s to understand sleep. Sleep studies started in 1937 with the discovery of the five successive sleep phases thanks to the electroencephalogram. The study of sleep in children is much more recent, and the literature is much less abundant than for adults. Only sick or hospitalized children were the subjects of extensive research. The first electroencephalographic recordings on children date from 1960, and they were only done on sick children. It was not until 1980 they recorded and filmed healthy children. Two methods are used to collect information on children's sleep: the sleep diary and altimetry. The technological progress will allow analyzing the rest of children, specifically in the future.

Scientists have presented two hypotheses to explain sleep. The first is that man, and his rhythm of life is adapted to the light. Although the human eye is familiar with darkness, it does not see as well by day as by night. Therefore, the night was synonymous with risk. It thus allowed the man to avoid the danger of nighttime, and that is why we sleep longer at night. The second hypothesis is that sleep allows man to recover from his physical activity during the day.

Sleep is a basic need for everyone. It allows the body to secrete growth hormones and white blood cells, which play a fundamental role in our immune system. Sleep also strengthens our neural circuits but also our cognitive capacities, such as memorization. Concentration also depends on the quality of sleep. Indeed, if the rest is respected, it allows better results in our activities.

Sleep functions are many, but memory is crucial for children. Sleep helps develop two types of memory:

- **Declarative memory:** consists of memorizing information in the verbal form, which can then be expressed by language.

- **Procedural memory:** allows the use and acquisition of motor skills such as walking, fine motor skills, etc.

During the day, the brain cannot store the information learned. Only a moment of rest allows our hippocampus to manage learning, transfer information, and delete it.

Sleep studies are becoming more and more precise. In 1959, the neurobiologist, Michel Jouvet discovered REM sleep. Indeed, the human brain is cyclical and composed of rhythms and cycles of rest. Sleep cycles are composed of slow sleep and REM sleep. The duration of a cycle is from 1h30 to 2h00 for the adult. The alternation of the day-night rhythm shapes our internal clock. Our period of sleep is continuously changing throughout life. During an adult sleep cycle, we can identify five sleep phases.

Sleep: C is a period in-between. The person is neither asleep nor completely awake. There are very few bodily movements.

Slow sleep:

- **Very light slow sleep** (phase I) and **light slow sleep** (phase II). Slow sleep happens when the person is calm and therefore sleeps. She can wake up if there is a sudden noise. During this time, the brain is active; dreams are logical and closer to real-life than of the imagination.

- **Slow/deep sleep** (phase III) is a very deep, **slow sleep** (phase IV). In this phase, the individual does not react to outside noises and is motionless. The face shows no expression, there are no eye movements, and mental activity is low. Breathing is slow and regular, and the muscle tone is the same as when awake.

REM sleep (phase V): The mental activity is very intense and is the same as a state of enlightenment. The face is expressive, breathing is rapid, and eye movements are visible. The body is hypotonic, and sometimes we have transient paralysis. C is, at this moment, the dream subject.

If a person wakes during this stage, he will manage to describe his dream very precisely. The individual dreams several times during the night, and the dream that is best remembered is that which occurs during the last sleep cycle.

Latency phase: After the succession of these phases and, therefore, the end of a complete cycle, the individual wakes up or begins a new sleep cycle.

CHAPTER TWO

Why is my toddler not sleeping?

When a child comes into the world, everything changes. You need to learn to adapt your circadian rhythm and to the rhythm of the toddler in a short time. The newborn is sleeping a lot but often waking up to eat as well. For this reason, the mother must learn to sleep in installments. Most of the babies switch between daytime and nighttime activities in the first months of life. But what if your child won't sleep at night? Constant lack of sleep and associated exhaustion have an adverse effect on the overall health of my mother. Why wake up your child? The likely reasons for that are here:

1. **Does not distinguish day from the night.**

When a child sleeps well during the day and wakes up often at night, he has not yet learned to differentiate between sleeping in the day and sleeping nightly.

We're recommending you! To keep the child from confusing daytime naps with nighttime sleep, it's worth placing him to sleep in a different place than at night, e.g., in a bassinette.

Do not darken the nap area when putting your toddler down for a nap during the day. Leave the blinds open or turn the radio down or close the window. Put your child in a bassinette during the day, instead of in his crib. Daytime has sound, light, and movement. The evening is when we wind-down from the day. Then dim the lights, whisper, and place your child in a cot that prevents vigorous movements.

2. There is no constant rhythm of the day.

The child must work at a specific speed of the day. A strategic nighttime strategy promotes the little one's understanding of what is happening around him. It gives him a sense of safety and calms him down. Daily routines govern the day; nightly routines govern the night.

If you want your child to sleep in day and night at certain times - teach him. When your toddler knows the rules and knows when it's time to nap, he won't protest. Evening rituals are a sign that the nightly resting time is approaching for the child. When your toddler remembers the order of activities and gets used to the plan, at certain times, he will have no problem falling asleep.

3. He's sad to be left alone.

You are the entire world to him. The youngster feels your closeness most of the day. You are feeding him, carrying him, wearing him, you are always beside him. A common reason why a child has trouble falling asleep is that the moment you place your baby in the crib, you disappear. How can it be fixed? Put a cot next to your bed. The child will sleep more peacefully, knowing you're close to him.

4. She is hungry.

Now and then, children fed on demand to eat appropriately. Slightly older babies (after six weeks of age) will eat for a bit longer, extending the meal cycles to 3-4 hours. It's normal for infants to need to be fed at night in the first months of life. A hungry baby doesn't sleep until his tummy is full. If your baby wakes up regularly, why not take him to bed and feed him lying there? Either nursing or bottle-feeding will work. The 6-month-old baby will sleep most evenings without eating any more.

5. They need a diaper change.

If the child doesn't want to sleep, then the explanation might be obvious - he has a wet diaper. You shouldn't wake up at night if you are using fine, absorbent diapers. But, no matter how absorbent the diapers are, if he has a bowel movement, change his diaper. Chafing is not pleasant, and is another reason for restless sleep.

6. He is too hot or too cold.

The optimal room temperature for the child should be around 20-22 ° C. The toddler can wake up if he's too hot or too cold. Don't wrap him too warmly, though. His method of thermoregulation continues to develop.

Don't forget! In a child's room, the optimum temperature is 20-22 during the day, 2 degrees less at night.

If you know your child doesn't like blankets and you're afraid it will get too cold, try putting him in a zipped sleeping bag. The child won't kick the blankets off, and you'll be sure he won't get cold.

7. Something hurts.

If a child doesn't want to sleep, and he or she wakes up crying soon after he or she sleeps, then there may be a warning that something is hurting. A taut body, a baby's bulging belly, screaming in the middle of the night, are common symptoms of colic.

If the child wakes up at night and they've grown out of colic, that may be a sign of teething. Gingival pain is so severe that holding them may not be enough at times. In these cases, gum numbing ointments that relieve pain may be used.

8. **He is uncomfortable.**

The baby wakes up occasionally because he's just tired. The reason may be a tag on clothing, too tight of a diaper, "biting" blanket, too soft, or too hard mattress. Check if the child's skin is irritated by the clothes, quilt, or cuddly toys.

9. **The sickness begins.**

If your baby is up and his nose is blocked, it might be the start of a cold. Children breathe primarily through the nose, so an infant's runny nose immediately wakes him out of sleep. After you've cleaned his nose, and the baby is still waking up and behaving differently than normal, this may mean the start of a cold.

10. **Because it was a day full of emotions!**

It can be hard to calm down when the child has encountered a lot of emotions during the day. Several experiences influence the state of the child in the evening. The child may need more time to calm down after a stressful day before falling asleep. Those days you can lengthen the bath a little, so your child can relax and calm down before you put him to sleep.

CHAPTER THREE

My baby doesn't sleep well - keys to help babies and toddlers sleep.

Sleep is one of the most significant human-health and development processes. When it is insufficient or inadequate, very diverse problems begin to emerge both in the person's physical health and in his psychological evolution. This is particularly important for babies and younger children, among many other reasons, since one of the functions of sleep is to stabilize the learning so quickly that the little ones do it continuously. It is, therefore, essential they have enough and restful sleep to develop well in all areas.

Sleep patterns differ with age (both in the number of hours of sleep and in their day-to-day distribution), and from one child to another. Therefore, instead of measuring it according to conventional criteria, it is necessary to be attentive to your baby's or your child's actions to see if it is difficult for him to fall asleep or if he is too tired or sleepy during the day, as anticipated at his era.

When sleep-related difficulties arise, an individualized evaluation is needed to find the most appropriate solution.

What are the most common causes of sleep difficulties in infants and young children?

Difficulty in identifying the days and nights: babies are not born knowing how to identify the right time to sleep, but this is something they learn with age when their habits are more accustomed to the day-night cycles. If you teach him to differentiate the nocturnal clues from daytime, you will help your child with this learning. Morning and midday are the best times to obtain sun, communicate, and play with him. The house should become quieter and darker at night, so avoid behaviors that agitate the child and even suggest more repetitive rituals to him, which will make sleeping easier for him.

Overstimulation at night: Stimulating the child too much at night is a common difficulty concerning the above. Sometimes this is because of the time when the parents return from work and can interact with him. This will, however, increase your level of activation and may interfere with your night sleep. Try to leave as much time as possible between moments of game and action, and activities of the night. Speak to him in a quiet and relaxed voice at night, preferably in dim light, and avoid distractions, games, or things that are of great interest to him.

Reacting too quickly: We may be concerned or even frightened when we hear a baby or a small child making noises at night, fearing that he may have choked or started crying. It's common for them to make little noises while they're sleeping, though, and if we go in their room right away, we can wake them up. Therefore, it is better to take a few seconds before going to see him before minor noises. We shouldn't wake him up unless it's essential, and if he wakes up, but he's quiet, it's better to wait until he's sleeping alone rather than communicating with him at the time.

Stimulate him as we try to calm him down: our efforts at calming our children sometimes have the opposite effect, either because we turn on the lights, speak to him loudly, or feel nervous about getting him to settle down and go back to bed. Do it softly, in low light, talk as little as possible, and don't make sudden gestures as you try to calm your child during the night. Do not bring games or other entertaining stimuli to your attention that help capture your attention and wake you up.

Bedtime isn't enough. Perhaps the time we put him to sleep is too early (so he won't be sleepy yet and won't want to sleep) or too late (so he might get irritable at bedtime and find it hard to sleep also). Pay attention to the signs of tiredness in your child and the time they usually sleep (or show signs of sleeping). It's better to take the period as a starting point, and slowly follow the sleep schedule you think is most suitable.

Nap too late. Taking a nap very late in the afternoon in children aged six months can make you get too close to bedtime at night and, therefore, not sleepy.

A hot bath in the evening. Before going to sleep, incorporating this routine will help the baby or child settle down and sleep more quickly, if this practice is a peaceful and non-stimulating moment for him.

Just don't be precise. Some parents, tired and irritated by the sleeping problems of their infant, are trying different conflicting approaches, without finding one that will work. When you want to apply a strategy, you need to be consistent with it for quite a few days, as it's the way your baby learns and adapts to the new patterns. Every day trying out a new method will lead to more uncertainty.

Health problems. Medical problems are a rare cause of sleep problems, but it is advisable to consult with a pediatrician to rule out possible physical disorders given their potential severity.

Schedule a sleep routine.

One of the best ways to get your child to sleep quickly is to introduce a routine 20 or 30 minutes before going to bed. It is about performing a series of rituals, every day, that involve calm, pleasant, and predictable activities so that the child associates this routine with the moment of sleep and prepares for it.

Some keys to carry out this ritual successfully are:

Enter quiet keys: the atmosphere of this moment must be different from the rest of the day. Use low light, move calmly, use a low tone of voice and a few words, etc.

It includes pleasant moments: a hot bath, reading a story, giving a massage. These are relaxing activities that can have a calming effect on your child and help you sleep peacefully.

Take advantage of the moment in which you are naturally sleepy: if we try to apply this routine at a time when the child is not tired, he will most likely resist falling asleep, thereby losing all the effectiveness of the previous ritual. Observe the moment you get naturally sleepy and start the routine 20 minutes before. Once the routine takes effect, and it is easy for you to fall asleep in this way, you can gradually advance or delay the time to go to sleep (10 or 15 minutes every several days).

Allow him to learn to fall asleep alone: if after this routine, take the child to his crib or his bed, and he will learn to fall asleep by himself and associate that context with a sleeping situation. On the contrary, if we allow him to sleep in other cases regularly (e.g., our arms), the child will not learn to fall asleep alone and will need your presence to go back to sleep when he wakes up in the middle of the night.

Even so, we agree that babies and young children's sleeping needs differ from one to the other and depend on age, so it is essential to respond to the needs and characteristics of each moment.

CHAPTER FOUR

Healthy sleep habits for your baby and child.

Sleep is a crucial aspect of health and wellbeing for your children. From birth, good sleep habits are learned.

Children who are not getting enough sleep may have difficulty getting through their day. They could have trouble falling asleep at night.

How much my child needs sleep?

Every single child is different. Some sleep a lot, and others sleep a lot less.

Babies (from birth to 4 months).

Newborns can sleep up to 18 hours a day, 3-4 hours a day. Waking up at night to eat is normal and healthy for them. When they get older, the child can stay awake for longer in the daytime and sleep longer in the evening.

Just like adults, babies need to know the right signs when it's time to sleep. If you're always putting your baby in his crib to sleep, for example, he'll know he's sleeping here. Your baby will eventually make the connection, even if he doesn't immediately understand.

Your baby will have developed more consistent sleeping habits a little after three months of age, and you will be able to establish a more daily napping schedule. Listen to the clues your baby shows. They'll let you know he's tired. Start a sleep journal, which will help you develop a regular sleep schedule.

It is good to establish a routine before naps. This routine can include a hug and a short story in a dark room.

Healthy sleep habits for your young baby:

- A child who is too tired will have more trouble sleeping. Eating helps your baby sleep better at night. Keeping him awake during the day will not help him sleep longer at night.

- Put your baby in bed while he is sleepy, but before he falls asleep. Be sure to place them on their back, in their bed, on a firm, flat surface, and avoid soft surfaces such as pillows and stuffed animals.

- There is nothing wrong with snuggling and rocking your baby. You cannot spoil a newborn baby by holding it in your arms.

- The pacifier can comfort your baby and help him fall asleep. However, wait until breastfeeding is well established before using it.

- Your baby will wake up at night. Give him a few minutes to go back to sleep alone before you go to see him.

- Avoid stimulating your baby when feeding and change his diaper overnight. Keep the lighting dim.

Babies (4 to 12 months).

Baby's sleep around 14 hours a day at this age but it may be common to sleep longer or less. At four months, most babies require three naps per day, one in the morning, one in the afternoon, and one in the early evening.

Your baby will probably go from three naps a day to two longer naps in the morning and afternoon, between the ages of six and 12 months. The needs of each baby are different. Many people take a 20-minute nap while others sleep for three hours or more.

Healthy Sleep Habits for Your Baby:

- Have a daily nap and bedtime routine where possible.

- Maintaining a consistent routine is essential. Many parents like using the same three elements: give him a warm bath of water, read him a book, and put him in bed.

- Try not to encourage your baby to sleep with his bottle. This habit helps the deterioration of the tooth.

- If your baby wakes up at night and cries around the age of 6 months, go and see him make sure everything's well, that he's neither too cold nor too hot, but don't get him out of his bed. Comfort him by stroking his brow or softly speaking to show him you are there. This will allow him to learn to comfort himself, which is necessary for him to learn to go back to sleep by himself.

Toddlers (1 to 2 years old).

Many babies sleep over 24 hours of 11 to 14 hours.

Safe Sleeping Habits for Toddler

- Maintaining a sleep schedule that your child recognizes is still vital. Habits set before age one are essential for your little one.

- During the day, stop naps too late, as they can interfere with nighttime sleep.

- Help your child calm down by telling them stories about half an hour before bedtime and leading them to calming activities.

- When your child protests, be gentle but firm.

- Keep your bedroom quiet, relaxed, and sleep-friendly, for example, using dim lighting.

- The music can be soothing and relaxing.

- In this period, transitional objects (such as a blanket or stuffed animal) sometimes take on significance.

Children (3 to 5 years old).

Usually, preschoolers sleep 10 to 13 hours a day. Around the age of three, your child will probably only have one nap a day, but many will take a second one. He may need a rest some days, but not others. Some children completely stop taking naps during this time. You can take advantage of the time spent in the nap, often after dinner, so that your child spends a quiet time reading and relaxing.

At this age, it is common for children to have certain sleep disorders and refuse to go to bed. They can also wake up at night because of night scares or nightmares.

Healthy Sleep Habits for Your Preschooler:

- Do not give your child drinks containing caffeine.

- Avoid screens before bedtime. Do not allow your child to have a tablet, TV, computer, or video game in their bedroom.

- Some children try to delay bedtime. Set limits, such as the number of books you will read to him, and make sure your child knows them.

- Tuck your child in by tightening the covers tightly to give your child a feeling of security.

- Don't ignore fears at bedtime. If your child has nightmares, reassure, and comfort him.

Some common sleep problems:

- Lack of sleep: Some children don't get enough sleep. If your child is difficult, irritable, or has trouble staying asleep at night, it may be because he is not napping long enough or going to bed too late.

- Separation problems: Your child may find it difficult to relax and fall asleep if he is disturbed by your absence. A very long hug before bedtime, a transitional object like a blanket or stuffed animal, or leaving the door open at night can help.

- Nightmares: Most children have nightmares at one time or another. Nightmares can occur after a stressful physical or emotional event or can be caused by fever. Your child can call you for comfort. Talk to him calmly, cuddle him, and reassure him.

When should I see my doctor?

- Loud snoring: If your child snores loudly regularly, he may have a problem.

- Sleepwalking: Sleepwalking is when a child wakes up partially during the night, but not entirely. He can sit in bed and repeat specific movements, such as rubbing his eyes. He can get out of bed and walk into his room. In general, if you talk to your child, they will not answer you. If your child is a sleepwalker, it is vital to make sure their environment is safe. Guide him gently to his bed without waking him. If the problem persists, contact your doctor.

- Night terrors: They are different from nightmares. Children who have night terrors cry without being able to control themselves, breathe quickly, and seem to be awake. If you wake them up, they may be confused and need a more extended period to calm down and go back to sleep. Night terrors occur mostly between the ages of 4 and 12, but they can start as early as 18 months of age. Most children end up getting rid of them on their own as they grow up, but if they persist, talk to your doctor.

What if my child regularly has trouble falling asleep?

Some children have trouble sleeping alone and can stay awake for long periods. This can be caused by spending too much time before bedtime in front of a television or by caffeine in soft drinks and energy drinks.

- If your child has long periods on computers, try limiting the screen time or excluding him from his routine.

- Do not allow your child to drink or eat products made from caffeine.

- Encourage relaxation before bedtime activities, such as reading, listening to quiet music, or having a calm conversation with your child about their day while lying with them on the bed.

If these are not responsible for your child's sleep problems, talk to your doctor about other ways to help him fall asleep on his own.

Baby Sleep: The Importance of Good Habits.

Not only do sleep disorders usually occur in adults, but children can also suffer from sleep problems and night awakenings.

What are the most common sleep disorders in children from birth to three years of age?

Parents most often consult me for trouble falling asleep and waking at night. The infant objects to bedtime, which has terrible family implications. Parents are drained, and this state of tiredness can lead to a variety of problems, depression, and a general family health disorder.

The most critical moment is around the age of two when the infant is gaining control and checking his parents ' boundaries. Bedtime is contradictory, and the setting of limits is essential.

What are the leading causes of these disorders?

The trigger is mostly in lousy behavior at bedtime for the difficulty of falling asleep, which is often related to night awakenings. Many parents get used to letting the child fall asleep in their arms or bed; others spend too much time with him before bedtime, putting him on a bottle to sleep or turning on the TV. In other cases, the cause lies in a search for intimacy with the parents, when the days are busy, and the child feels like a "package" transported from the nanny to the house and then to bed, without having spent quiet time with his parents.

Family stress, excessively long naps, or even parental lack of authority can also interrupt the child's sleep. Yet symptoms such as hallucinations, night terrors, restless sleep, snoring, and falling asleep in an odd position can sometimes mask sleep apnea problems.

Among other things, it is normal for the child to sleep poorly in certain situations: during his first year of life, the structure of his sleep changes significantly, awakenings for physiological causes are frequent. If he's sick, if the room temperature isn't ideal, and if he's going through a transition time that's distracting him, his sleep will be weak.

What can parents do to avoid poor sleep, or handle it?

Above all, they shouldn't worry as sleep disorders rarely have implications for their development and mental functioning in a healthy child. This typically compensates for breaks and naps during the day.

If the troubles persist and disturb the whole family, you should talk to a specialist during a dedicated consultation, as suggested by researchers. The answer to each problem is individual, on a case-by-case basis. But among the techniques that give good results, there is the 5-10-15 rule. Once the baby is lying down, if he starts to cry, the parents must wait five minutes and then go and reassure him by explaining to him, without touching him, that "it's night, everything is fine in the house, it's time to sleep." If necessary, the operation should be repeated after ten and then 15 minutes. In general, this technique works after 2-3 days because the child feels the determination of his parents.

From 5-6 months, he must learn to fall asleep alone and in bed. To achieve this, respecting a sleep ritual that reassures the child is essential. You also need to learn to spot the signs of sleep and go to bed as soon as they appear. The baby should not get into the habit of falling asleep with a human presence.

CHAPTER FIVE

Naps.

Until the age of about three months, we do not define the baby's sleep by speaking of "naps." Indeed, until then, the baby spends a lot of time sleeping. The waking time is mainly intended for meals. At this age, also, the baby begins to distinguish day and night. This keeps the baby awake longer during the day and sleeps for more hours at night. C is currently that we talk about naps for babies.

For nine months, specialists recommended that the baby sleeps for about fifteen hours (half-past eleven at night and three and a half hours in two naps). For this age group, the sleep time required at night will be the same until the age of eight. Between nine and twelve months, the nap at the end of the afternoon begins to disappear. If the latter continues to be present, it is because the rest at the start of the afternoon is not long enough.

The daytime nap - how to make it a ritual?

For a child, it's not just night sleep that is significant. The short naps that occur over the day are equally important.

These occur several times, and then several times during the day, depending on the infant's age. The brain begins a period of tremendous operation when the body of the toddler is asleep. It organizes information, establishes and strengthens nerve connections during deep sleep (REM-phase characterized by rapid eye movements). The body releases growth hormones during the shallow sleep phase, regenerates tissues, heals wounds, and strengthens the immune system.

Let's not hide that the nap time for the child is also a precious moment for the parent - a moment of relaxation, a respite from the child's bustle (and often the period when they can take care of other housework).

These claims recommend supplying the infant with the best conditions for a part of daily sleep: day and night. What does that mean, and how do you do that?

- **Between Nap and Sleep.**

Ultrasounds show that a baby sleeps a lot in the womb. Even during childbirth, she is in a kind of half-sleep, from which the most vigorous contractions often only force them out.

The infant also often goes between sleep and wakefulness in the first days of life. Many newborns then sleep almost without a break, while others sleep just about a dozen or so hours a day. Some researchers believe that during the genetically programmed day is, children tend to take a short or long nap, and parents' impact on the time and length of sleep in such a small child is very minimal.

At about three months of age, wakefulness gradually emerges from sleep. Then the toddler sleeps even three or four times a day. These naps last from several dozen minutes to over three hours. Some babies fall asleep after each feeding. However, some sleep before noon, after lunch, take a short, hour nap, and then have a significantly more extended period of activity in the afternoon.

- **Age and Dreaming.**

The six-month-old baby cuts down to only two naps during the day. His bedtime ceases to depend strictly on the time of eating (a full stomach does not automatically cause drowsiness; the baby wakes up not because he is hungry but because he has just gotten enough sleep). The one-year-old child usually sleeps once or twice during the day: about an hour before noon and one to three hours in the afternoon.

Between the first and second years of life, most children give up a morning nap. Then the best time to sleep during the day is early afternoon. A nap usually lasts about two hours. It is worth remembering, however, that it should not start later than at three or four in the afternoon so that the toddler does not have trouble falling asleep in the evening. At least three to four hours should elapse between waking up and bedtime.

- **Rhythm Issue.**

We do not influence the matter of the "genetic tendency to sleep," as well as on the maturation of the toddler and natural, gradual growing out of frequent and long naps.

What we have is to make it easier for the child to calm down, set a constant rhythm of the day, and introduce specific habits that are to signal him that it is time to sleep and rest. How does it look in practice?

First, try to put it to sleep at about the same time. Secondly, the baby must fall asleep during the day, where at night (this, in turn, will make it easier for him to fall asleep in the evening), i.e., most often in his cot. Thirdly, it is best for the sleeping place to be in a quiet and peaceful corner of the house, which will help your child calm down.

However, the introduction of such habits does not always end with results or work as fast as we would like.

If a several-month-old baby has chosen a vigorous time of day for you to watch, e.g., morning, instead of getting frustrated, try to move it gradually.

- **With Full Belly.**

During the first months of life, the toddler falls asleep properly with each feeding. This is determined not only by the soothing warmth and closeness of my mother but also by the feeling of satiety, which affects the sense of drowsiness. So when a baby wakes up from a morning nap, it's worth feeding him. This will probably put him to sleep again, and then the next meal will come later.

After a few days, the child will get used to the long morning sleep and longer awake in the afternoon. An older baby's full stomach is no longer enough to take a long nap (because it is much harder to fill it). A six-month-old child wakes up when he is hungry. His bedtime ceases to depend strictly on the time of eating.

However, it is worth thinking about more filling meals before bedtime, so that the feeling of satiety lasts longer. Porridges or gruel fulfill this task well. Their additional advantage is that they are very quickly and easily prepared. For a hungry and sleepy toddler, as well as for his mother or father, every minute when preparing a meal is at a premium.

Lesson Sleeping A.

A newborn baby can sleep anywhere. However, when he is two or three months old, external stimuli (noise, harsh light) may prevent him from falling asleep. This is the moment when you can try to get your child to fall asleep on their own. For many parents, however, this is a difficult task, especially for mothers who have become accustomed to putting the toddler to sleep.

It is worth trying to put the baby to sleep when he is not asleep; do not put him to sleep on his hands or by the breast. In return, you can introduce another ritual: put the baby in a cot, cover the curtains, sit for a moment, humming the lullaby, or a pat on the back. An older baby can be given a pacifier or cuddly toy. If the toddler cries, instead of taking him your arms, it is better to investigate the cot and calm him down, speaking to him in a gentle voice. Younger infants generally agree more quickly with the new ritual and fall asleep without too much protest on the second or third day.

This first lesson, though it seems complicated, is essential. Because there is a chance that thanks to her, the toddler will have less trouble falling asleep in the future, and when he wakes up at night (which happens quite often to children), he will be able to fall back to sleep without putting the whole house on his feet.

Sleeping Through the Night.

It is also important to note what is actually "sleeping through." (For the tired, maybe even sleepless parents, it may not be the holy grail you imagined.)

A baby is known to sleep through the night when, in one stretch, they sleep six — yes, just six — hours. Perhaps your baby is sleeping through the night already, and you didn't realize it. Do not worry. It may not feel like it (as time appears to feel very slow in the throes of infant raising and sleep training), but soon enough, your child will be sleeping for more significant periods. It may take months to get there, but your child's overnight sleep will begin to lengthen and eventually reach on average from 10 to 12 hours or more a night.

Naptime and Bedtime Routines.

If you believe the naps and nighttime sleep of your child need to be retooled, there are simple ways of instituting improvement that can pay off in significant ways. Just don't expect your child to experience immediate growth or positive, tear-free cooperation. Each parent has their level of comfort in different approaches to try, and how much self-sufficiency they allow for their child. Follow your instincts to make decisions about what's right for your family. Here are some potential methods for dealing with sleep improvement, as well as general implementation tips to help you move towards more restful nights.

- Gently make changes. For instance, if you try to drop from four naps a day to two, lose one nap at a time, allowing your baby time to adapt to the new pattern.

- Aim to maintain similar bedtime and naptime routines. Bring your baby down for a nap, for example, in the same place they're supposed to sleep at night. It helps establish comfort and confirms that this is the place to sleep.

- Don't allow newborns to become habits. Young infants are likely to be unprepared for scheduled naps and sleep in irregular patterns. This is natural and one that should be predicted.

- Pay attention to the signs of your baby's fatigue— they try to pin you in when they need to sleep.

- At first sign of tiredness, try to place your child down. It's important not to wait until your baby is exhausted full-blown, which tends to lead to comfortable sleep, and less.

- Build a schedule to which you can confirm, to timing that fits well in your day. For example, don't plan to get your baby down for a nap around the same time they need to pick up their sibling for pre-school.

- Be versatile (including your child and yourself). If you can't exactly stick to your routine, you might be able to sneak into the car seat or stroller in naptime if you need to be on the go or in a child carrier if your little one isn't going to settle on their own.

- Try to lie down with your baby for a nap (and maybe to catch yourself a nap).

CHAPTER SIX

Reasons why your baby is waking at night and won't sleep.

One of the most common problems parents try to help their baby solve is a baby who wakes at night. One move in learning how to make a night of baby sleep better at night is to understand better why a baby wakes up at night.

1. Your baby has a sleep association.

"Sleep association" is also known as "sleep aids" or "crutches," meaning that your baby has a specific item or way they've been conditioned to believe they "need" to fall asleep. That will be a pacifier, bottle feeding, or breastfeeding for many babies to sleep. This can be some movement for other babies, such as rocking, bouncing, walking, or a ride in the car. Many babies with higher needs will come to rely on a variety of sleep crutches, like bouncing with a pacifier.

The baby's age and the form of sleep relationship are the two factors that must be taken into account when deciding the best course of action to be taken to help encourage a baby to fall asleep alone and break his dependence on his sleeping crutch. It's also a good idea to keep the personality of the baby in mind when developing a sleep training program.

2. New Developmental Milestones.

Learning how your baby crawls, raises, walks, and speaks are all developmental milestones that can interfere with your baby's night sleep and nap times. The main thing to keep in mind about sleep disruptions due to developmental milestones is that if your baby doesn't seem to be learning new skills, it doesn't mean that they haven't mastered them yet.

Although a developmental milestone that temporarily interferes with sleep improvement, it does not mean that your baby is still not learning sleep habits when you stay consistent with sleep training. If your baby reaches an age where she can learn how to go back to sleep by herself, night waking becomes less frequent and is much less stressful for the whole family.

3. Your Baby is Teething.

It may feel like your baby has been teething for two years continuously, particularly when many babies experience teething problems long before a tooth even breaks out. If teething seems to make your baby wake up more than a night, it can be challenging to know how to handle it and continue to teach your baby how to sleep well. Parents may ask, "Is my baby in pain?" "Is that why my baby wakes all night? "Often a baby-waking due to teething is a temporary phase in which a baby returns to their regular sleeping patterns until they feel better as long as the parents have tried to stay consistent with putting the baby to sleep as they did before teething and during the teething process.

4. Baby is hungry.

Most parents are advised that after a certain age, their baby shouldn't need a nighttime feeding. This could be so if each baby is the same and has the same needs. This is is not the case. For average, a lot of babies at six months of age will still need feeding or two. It's essential to keep in mind that for a baby with a small tummy to go without eating 11-13 hours is a long time. A night-waking baby out of hunger can still be fed without having a feeding sleep connection, and often a night-time feed is just what a baby needs to keep sleeping through the rest of the night.

5. Babies are human too.

While it's true that most babies thrive on a regular schedule and routine, parents can sometimes lose perspective and get upset about why their baby doesn't sleep the same day. Babies are humans too, not robots. We will have some unpredictability about them, their personality, their interests, and their needs. Many babies do sleep and wake like clockwork, but there are just as many who do not. As a parent may not be hungry every day at the same time, a baby may not sleep at the same time every night. Babies, just like everyone else, will have good days to sleep and bad days.

There are many reasons why a baby will wake up at night and have trouble with the baby's sleep. Try to understand why your baby would wake up at night and then work to find a solution, whether it's a temporary relief during a stressful process or weaning her from a sleep association. When babies grow, they can develop, and their ability to learn and understand dramatically increases. The same will be true concerning their sleep habits, so it is best to try to be versatile and accommodating yet consistent when teaching your baby how to sleep better.

How to help the baby sleep through the night.

Develop a rhythm.

Newborns sleep 16 or more hours per day, but generally in stretches of a few hours at a time. Although the sleep pattern may be variable at first, it will be regularized as the baby matures and can spend more time between meals.

By 3 or 4 months of age, many babies sleep for at least five hours straight. At some point during the first year of life — all babies are different — you will begin to sleep about 10 hours a night.

Make the baby sleep in your room.

Ideally, the baby will sleep in your room with you, but only in a crib, bassinet, or other structure designed for babies for at least six months and, if possible, for up to a year. This can reduce the risk of sudden infant death syndrome.

Adult beds are not safe for babies. The baby can get caught and suffocate between the slats of the headboard, or in the spaces between the mattress and the bed structure, or the mattress and the wall. A baby can also suffocate if a sleeping parent moves by accident and covers the baby's nose and mouth.

How to encourage good sleep habits.

During the first months, feeding in the middle of the night will inevitably interrupt the sleep of both parents and babies, but it is never too early to help your baby begin to sleep well. Keep the following tips in mind:

- **Follow a regular and relaxing bedtime routine**. Nighttime overstimulation will make it difficult for your baby to settle down to sleep. Once you leave the room, run a bath, kissing, singing, listening to quiet music or reading, with a clearly defined endpoint. Continue those tasks in a quiet room with dim lighting until your baby is too tired to stay awake.

- **When sleepy, take the baby to bed but wake them up**. This will help your baby relate the bed to the falling asleep process. Remember to put the baby on his back and remove the covers and other soft items from the crib.

- **Give your child some time to calm down.** Once you find a comfortable position and fall asleep, your baby may have tantrums or scream. If he doesn't stop crying, check on him to see that he's well, tell him something to calm him down, and leave the room. The baby may need your calming presence to get asleep.

- **Consider giving him a pacifier.** If your baby is having trouble calming down, then a pacifier might be enough. Indeed, research suggests that using a pacifier during sleep helps to reduce the risk of sudden death syndrome among infants.

- **It provides quiet night care.** Use dim lighting, soft voice, and relaxed gestures when you need to attend or feed your baby during the night. This will tell your baby it's time to sleep and not play.

- **Respect preferences for your baby**. You may want to change the habits and schedules based on these typical trends if your baby is a night owl or an early bird.

CHAPTER SEVEN

How do parental involvement and baby sleep training work together?

Parents who practice or want to practice parenting attachment often struggle with the notions of how to train their baby to sleep and how to help their baby sleep through the night. One of the main principles of attachment parenting fosters the belief that sleep training techniques can have adverse psychological and physiological effects on the child, primarily by crying it out. Co-sleeping is strongly encouraged with attachment parenting to ensure that baby needs are met at night, including helping to soothe them at night when they wake up.

The common misconception is that sleep training means just making the baby cry it out to learn how to soothe themselves and put themselves to sleep. It is not real. There are other ways to make your baby or toddler sleep through the night and learn how to fall asleep by themselves.

Attachment parenting components are designed to help babies and parents develop strong and healthy relationships in part by tuning in and responding appropriately to what babies need—helping your baby learn how to sleep and have healthy sleep patterns is part of tailoring a baby's needs. Having your baby sleep through the night or having your baby sleep longer is sensitive to the need for sleep that your baby has. It's essential also to remember that not all babies are the same.

Babies ' various temperaments will play a part in how well a form of sleep training can perform. A no-cry solution to sleep can often be more useful for babies with a more persistent or strong-willed temperament.

Parents who practice parenting with attachment are very passionate about this parenting style. Many people will, however, accept that any kind of parenting that encourages healthy and positive relationships is suitable for babies and families. A growing family needs to find out what works for them, and this means teaching their baby to sleep for some families even as they practice parenting with attachment. Sleep training should take a variety of parenting styles into account, including parental attachment.

Sleep training should NOT involve regulated crying or crying out, or any other combination of it. Attachment parents potty train (mostly the baby-led), so why can't you sleep train? The obvious difference between potty training and sleep training is that potty training usually occurs when the child is a toddler, and at a younger age, sleep training will take place. If you can gently train potty, though, you can also lightly sleep train. If you understand the mechanics of sleep associations, then asleep coaching program can be developed which does not include leaving the baby to cry out.

But it can be unrealistic to expect no crying when your baby is learning how to fall asleep on its own, but you never have to leave your baby alone. Babies cry to express a need, and often they weep because they are upset that they cannot sleep or that they don't get enough sleep. Some cries will help make babies sleep better. Babies often need to gain the confidence to think they can fall asleep without your help.

This may mean you have to give your child the room to develop safe sleeping habits without breastfeeding, soothing or rocking the crutches to sleep. While your baby is crying during sleep training, it's ok to stay close to support during the transition. A baby who is not yet self-reassuring to sleep does not necessarily mean that if he can learn and practice this ability, he cannot self-reassure.

If mom and baby suffer from sleep deprivation, then sleep training is always worth a try, and you can continuously re-evaluate if your strategy is not going well. There is hope that even when you're "attachment parenting," you can make a difference in your and your baby's life by "sleep coaching."

CHAPTER EIGHT

Beds For Toddler - Tips On Selecting A Right Bed.

A child bed helps a child make the transition from a crib to an adult bed. They're tiny but cute and cozy enough for the child to sleep in. Toddler beds should be low in height to ensure safety for an infant. We can have four-sided railings. When the bed is in use, those railings can be rolled out.

Toddler beds come in enchanting styles and a wide variety. We put consistency and fun together and will encourage every child to go to bed. Picture your child jumping into a bed shaped like a toy train with bells and whistles, and books and toys storage space. Little boys love beds in the form of cars, trucks, and motorbikes. Any of these would make your child want to give up his crib.

During the day, a person's wellbeing depends on the quality of the sleep. For a child, it's essential not only to sleep but also the quality of the bed furniture, mattresses, and fabrics. Experienced parents know it's a difficult job to choose a bed for a child. Many considerations must be considered, focusing on many choices related to operating conditions.

Because the choice should be taken seriously.

Parents tend to be pleased with a range of children's furniture. But conscientious parents should pay attention not only to the colored image but also to the consistency, the origin of the content. The unscrupulous manufacturers will make beds using sterile or even radioactive material.

The original design does not state the bed's functionality. If the child falls out of bed during sleep, this can have a wide range of behavioral, emotional, and mental implications. The design must, therefore, be unique but also safe.

Mattresses and models of beds should conform to the child's anatomical properties. In some cases, certain products are not considered by the manufacturer. Over time a child may experience scoliosis, the removal of internal organs. These are direct threats to children's health.

The choice of beds for children's needs to be approached carefully. Any information will affect the child's health and wellbeing during the active growth period.

Conditional beds can be classified into several types:

- Manufacture cots and cribs for the smallest manufacturers.

- The most famous up to now is the classic version of the hull style.

- To families with many children or small space in the home, a bunk bed may be a child's is the best option.

- The transforming beds are multifunctional structures, which include a bed, a desk, a play area, and multiple shelves.

- A children's loft bed is a choice for teenagers who want comfortable having their own space.

There are several modifications to the types presented which suggest the presence of auxiliary structures.

What you should pay attention to when choosing.

The age characteristics of the crumbs usually decide the bed for the infant. First, you should be paying attention to the cabinet furniture parameters. Typically, each model will be determined by a small consumer's age and parameters.

All the aspects related to the child's behavior are worth considering. If it turns at night, a model of furniture with sides is better to buy. When a child frequently gets up at night in the bathroom, the bed must be able to be adapted to these circumstances.

The product's presentation may be fine, but it is best to ask the seller for standard certificates.

- Permit for this company to produce children's furniture.

- Confirm the material quality as well as the product itself.

- Establishes all applicable regulations concerning insurance and grievances.

The certificate, of course, does not provide the perfect bed condition. In any case, a bed should be comfortable and not just appealing for an infant. The child's interests should be considered in the selection process, but no less consideration should be paid to secondary nuances.

What should be considered in the selection process?

In addition to the main points at the time of purchase, it is worth considering the minor features of the structures.

When you choose to follow a few simple rules:

- Choose wooden furniture.

- The design should not be sharp elements or corners.

- The textile component should be made of natural material.

- The children's bunk bed should be secure and reliable.

- There should be no bolts, strips, other items that a child can tear or unscrew.

A bed for two children does not have to be a bunk bed. Recently, two-bed trundle beds are accessible.

Choose a cot for a newborn.

Each bed for a child must correspond to his age. For newborns, various models of cribs, cribs, beds. The variety is due to the different functionality of the sleep device.

Types of beds for babies:

- Crib beds are especially popular with modern parents. The furniture can be equipped with a mechanical device to recreate an absolute amplitude of the swing. A simple option is a manual version for the swing.

- Cot with drawers. A simple bed located at the bottom of the boxes for things. Such models are relevant in small apartments.

- Cradle with built-in dressing room, chest of drawers, and open shelves. This hybrid furniture is multifunctional and very comfortable to use. Combine different elements of the space arrangement for the child.

- Arena bed. The real option for active children and busy parents will help save space in the apartment. High shelves allow the crumbs to play and sleep at the same time without endangering the life of the child.

Other features include shapes, sizes, colors, and materials. Additional equipment is a marketing tool for increasing sales.

When is it a Good Time to Move Toddlers to a Bed?

Originally the word bed is the place where a person sleeps. A bed wasn't much more than a hole in the ground in the beginning. The first kind of baby beds were cradles, and they were compact and well suited for an infant. Children's beds have a rich history. When a baby's news was arriving, they were more than certainly one of the first pieces of furniture brought into a house.

As homes grew larger during the 1800s, the baby crib came to be as they could accommodate a growing child's needs. Usually, they were handmade and then passed from child to child. Baby beds were also passed on to babies of newer generations, as they were most likely made from the area's sturdy wood.

When is the time to get your baby out of its cradle or crib?

You should move the baby to the larger bed when you notice your baby is outgrowing its crib. Most babies almost instantly take to sleep in a big bed, instead of sleeping in their crib. To infants and smaller children, a crib is made. There is no hard-fast procedure to move a baby out of a cradle and into a bassinet for a specific time.

In their third month, cradles generally become too small for a baby. You may wish to move the baby into a crib at this time to facilitate restful sleep. If your baby grows out of her cradle, now is the time to move him or her into the crib.

Babies grow and eventually begin to move about; if your baby moves in the bassinet, it can become dangerous for the infant. Because small children do not understand the consequences of gravity, and if the bassinet flips over, they cannot prevent themselves from falling.

Remember not to place any pillows or stuffed toys with your child in the crib, as they may pose the risk of succumbing to the SIDS syndrome of sudden infant death. When you leave pillows and toys in an infant's bed, they may smother to death. In your selection of a baby bed, you should be very careful so that you do not endanger your child while trying to care for it properly.

Through teaching it to enjoy the different beds, you will make the change from a cradle to a crib much easier for your infant.

How to Make the Transition to a Toddler Bed.

Once you've decided it's time to move your child to a baby bed, it's essential how you go about it. For a child, this is a significant change and can be very overwhelming. Here are some ideas and tips which hopefully will help you make your child as painless as possible.

Allow your child to participate in the decision to move into the new bed and help pick it up if possible. If you already have the bed and you don't have an option to buy a new one, then consider letting your child pick new sheets to cover them. This will make their bed more at heart and make the transition more meaningful for them.

Once you have the childbed, set it up for several weeks in the child's room before you move them in. This will give them a chance to get used to it, so it doesn't seem so new. If you need to, you can even get the child into the child's bed every night as part of the bedtime routine and lie there for a while. Perhaps while you're reading them a novel, and then, when you sleep, you shift them into their crib.

To reduce the actual amount of change, move everything possible from the crib into the toddler bed. You should choose to have them take their daytime naps in the bed but still sleep at night in their crib. When you're finally ready to start using the baby bed full time, you should take the crib down and move the baby bed to the same room location to ease the transition.

Patience is the order of the day, especially if your child is reluctant to give up the crib. Many children take their new big boy or girl bed without doubts, but it is a challenging change for many. Try not to do this at the same time, as there are other changes in your children's lives, whether they are just starting potty training, changing the daycare center, or adding a new family member.

Whatever you do, your child may not be ready for this move, so you need to be patient and wait a couple of months to try it again.

CHAPTER NINE

Getting Your Toddler to Sleep in Their Own Bed.

Most children feel happy and safe sleeping with their parents, but obviously, this situation can not last forever. You would finally want your child to learn to sleep in his crib. Follow the steps we are taking to make the transition as easy as possible.

1. **Prepare for the transition:**

Pick the right timing. Recall that teaching a young child to sleep alone is easier than changing an existing pattern in an older child, so consider starting as soon as you're able. Nevertheless, the goal would be to teach your child in a relatively peaceful and uncomplicated time to sleep in his bed-not when your life is full, or when the child is already facing other significant changes.

- Whether you intend on traveling or heading into the near future, it's best to wait. You won't be able to keep the new routine in such a stressful moment, and it would be difficult for a small child to have too many changes together.

- If your child is sick or faces other sleep-related issues (such as nightmares or fears of the night), it is equally best to wait until these problems have been resolved.

- If your child is already in the middle of another significant transition process (such as weaning him, training him to do without a pacifier or using a potty, or preparing to take him to kindergarten or kindergarten), consider postponing the transition from Latvian to the cot for your parents. Such changes are challenging for young children and focusing them all at the same time wouldn't be a good idea.

Talk the matter to your partner. Tell them about your intention to teach the child to sleep in his bed, if you have a partner. When faced with mutual support from both parents, the transition process will be much simpler (and less stressful). If your partner is firmly convinced that this move is still too early, don't try to force the decision.

Get your child ready for the transition. Explain what you expect from him and present the change in a cheerful and positive manner-as an exciting step that demonstrates how great and independent, he is.

Involve your child in bedroom preparedness. If you buy the sheets for his cot, take it with you and maybe let him choose a new toy or a special stuffed toy with which to sleep.

Practice naps during the day. Have your child take a bedtime nap in the afternoon. So, in a less stressful moment, he'll learn to associate it with the sleeping action.

2. **Bring your child to sleep in his bed:**

Keep unchanged the other activities that make up the bedtime routine. If you've already set up a daily routine to put your child in bed-such as bathing, putting on pajamas, eating a snack, reading the bedtime story, brushing your teeth, and then going to bed-keep every part of this routine unchanged except where you're going to put it to sleep. That way, even in the face of a significant change, the child's sense of stability will remain intact.

Let's be optimistic. Tell your child that it's an exciting change to sleep alone and make sure he knows you're proud of how significant and confident he gets. Tell him how much more room he'll have in his new bed and remind him of everything you've specifically chosen together for this moment, like the sheet set and the new toy.

Take a regular check of your children. Your baby can feel anxious, especially on the first night. Wish him goodnight with a relaxed display, give him a hug and a kiss, and then leave the room. If he's distraught, come back to him every ten minutes or so to briefly reassure him. If required, repeat this process.

Glory to your children. If he goes to sleep alone without getting a tantrum, overcoming his nervousness, or sleeping in his bed all night, then the next morning, congratulating him and praising him for how good he was. Positive reinforcement is of great assistance to the change.

3. **Manage His Resistance:**

Keep quiet. Most children scream and pleading for their parents to return to their cribs. All this is natural, so don't want to get upset. If your child sees you get angry, the situation gets worse.

Be decisive. Don't give in to tears and whining; if you do, your child will learn to manipulate you to get what he wants. If he is weeping and moaning in his room, check it out regularly, soothing him with a few words of comfort; when he wants to get out of bed, bring him back.

- Do not make exceptions. When you take a break from perpetrating this daily routine, perhaps because your child is sick or because he's had a bad dream, you're only going to confuse him and, as a result, he's going to offer even more change resistance.

- In these cases, it can be tough for a parent not to give in. You will probably feel like your child is being handled too cold or driven away, but if he sees you being positive, he will eventually feel less upset and more comfortable. Use a soft and affectionate tone and let your child know you're nearby, but don't give in and feel guilty about it.

Try to understand why it is that your child refuses. If she keeps crying, try to understand why. Try speaking to him during the day, when it is obvious. If you see that being with you at night is just stubbornness and the impulse, keep on keeping yourself optimistic and persistent in continuing the transition. If, on the other hand, you see that this is mostly a question of night fears-fear of the dark or monsters-you might be able to solve the issue by leaving a light on for the night and doing some practice of "monster-chasing."

Note also the possibility of proposing a more radical change. If your child tries to fight, then you can try sitting in his bedroom before he sleeps. After a few nights, step a little further away, close to the door. After a while, go outside the room to the hall.

Reward your child for his advances. You may be able to use a sticky sticker notebook or another system of rewards to encourage him to sleep in his bedroom.

Secrets of Having Sweet Sleeping Babies All Night Long.

The baby needs to be raised and trained the first time a sleeping baby sleeps all night. Children learn instinctively as well as their personal experience and adapt to their parents' lifestyle. Being a human is a busy experience, primarily if the offspring depends on your needs. No wonder many parents are tired and wanting rest at the end of the day.

Here are some tips to help your baby sleep and fall asleep.

- Start by keeping the baby busy throughout the day, unless you intend to sleep while the baby snuffs. This is an excellent idea for new mothers since; this is the healing time for the body as well. Speaking, singing, and playing with your child will keep them engaged as they learn, develop, and explore their surroundings. Just make sure it isn't a long nap while napping, as it will mess with the baby being able to sleep for the whole night.

- Much will attract the baby's attention, including mobiles, sounds, and light patterns. To raise a child who sleeps despite the noise, they must become used to it. It began in embryo for them; continue its use after the child arrives. Doing so won't limit you to being quieter than mice, so you don't wake the boy. It should suffice to click the telephone ringer down or off. On the other hand, you can be as pretty as possible and hope the baby stays asleep for the entire night. White noise appears to help minimize other household noises; you can promote sweet dreams for your child by merely turning a fan on low or using calming sound effect recordings.

- You may want to do some research on their use before using a pacifier to get your baby to go to sleep and sleep all night long, as well as remember the times the baby loses the pacifier when attempting to go to sleep or sleep all night long. Many children, on the other hand, can take a pacifier, and many others won't.

- Sleeping arrangements are a personal choice; however, training a baby to sleep in his bed is best. It is restful for everyone to be able to lie down, stretch out while going to sleep and sleep through the night. You just put the child in their rooms, just as they are about to go to sleep. Doing so allows them to take advantage of the environment as well as not get nervous while waking up somewhere I don't know.

- Take turns to get the baby to sleep in the night. Of course, both parents get up to see their new baby while keeping their partner company, but taking turns is better for everyone.

- Allowing others to support you when you are exhausted and need rest is a beautiful idea, as well as providing your baby with excellent opportunities to grow in their family structure and climate.

- Keep in mind that a baby will wake up many times during the night because they're hungry. When you lay down to sleep, if you feed them, they will be full and more likely to continue to sleep through the night.

CHAPTER TEN

Positive Discipline Techniques for Children.

In general, education methods are rooted in the use of punitive disciplines based on punishment, something that causes adverse effects. When looking for other alternatives, the parents go to the other extreme and give the child an excessive permissiveness.

The use of these methods so authoritarian or so permissive is given by the daily fatigue and monotony of the routines suffered by parents and makes them unable to stop to think if there are other ways of education.

As an effective alternative to these two educational models, positive discipline emerges. This is based on collaboration by respecting the child's responsibility and autonomy in love, in freedom of action, in the involvement of children, and the development of the child healthily and happily. Also, from this model, there are no wrong or good children, but good and bad behavior.

What is positive discipline?

The purpose of this type of education is for children to understand the rules that will provide them with security. This discipline should not be interpreted as an imposition of these norms, but as a means by which the child develops healthily and happily and as something that teaches them the way to be responsible for their actions and that every effort has a consequence. That also serves to learn the appropriate way to know how to behave and act in each situation.

In this way, with the positive discipline, it is sought to favor the maturation of children so that in the future, they are responsible, autonomous, and happy.

Techniques to educate children with positive discipline.

To teach from this model, we must remember that the use of physical and verbal punishments must be avoided and away from the imposition of norms and guidelines. Since the child must learn and not obey. Some positive discipline techniques are as follows:

- ***Praise what you like.*** Ponder, count, and relive those moments when the child behaves well. They are a way to reinforce the behaviors that you want to repeat.

- ***Give routines.*** Setting usual rules will prevent unwanted behavior. If, for example, the child knows that after playing he must pick up, he makes him understand that if one day he does not keep the toys he will be misbehaving and this will have consequences that he does not like and that he will have to assume. So, try to do well.

- ***Adult control.*** Bad behavior can be described as a "badly made" attention call. The child understands that you spend more time when adopting positions of this type. Do not pay attention when the child behaves unacceptably, instead of arguing with him. This way, you will learn that there are better ways to communicate. There are times when there is a tense situation, and you know that what you have done is very bad. It's hard to keep calm, but you must think that what we don't want them to do next should not be done in front of the child. Try to leave the place where your little one is or try to do relaxation exercises. Wait to have calmed down and come back in

- ***Ask instead of ordering.*** Thus, we ensure that the child knows the answer, and we give him the freedom to do things or not knowing the consequences of his actions. In this way, the child learns to behave and not to obey blindly. For example, what do we have to do now? And let the child respond.

- **Advance notice.** Before the end of the activity you are doing, tell him and remind him what is coming so that he does not catch you.

- ***Give behavioral options.*** Give them to choose the order in which they want to do the tasks they must perform. For example, do you prefer to shower before or after dinner?

- ***Rewards table.*** Setting clear limits and rules in writing can make the child see clearly that several well-done actions are reinforced.

- ***The example of the parents.*** It is the best technique of positive discipline. Children imitate all the behaviors that attract their attention if there are no other alternatives, so parents must act consistently to serve as a model for their children.

How to Promote Self-Discipline In Children?

The most appropriate method to promote self-discipline in children is the method of natural and logical consequences. It means that the child chooses one among several alternatives and experiences the result of his choice. The natural result of promoting self-discipline is all that allows us to learn what will happen naturally if we have certain behaviors. For example, if I tell my children that they must brush their teeth every day is not discipline. So how do we promote self-discipline in children?

When they grow up, they will get many cavities, and they will have to go to the dentist, the preschool child cannot understand something very well that is probably going to happen when they're old. There are natural consequences that we cannot use in our children, and that is why we have to collect a logical result, from here and now: "If you want to be in the classroom, and you throw the ball which you're not supposed to do, I take it away from you." That is telling him once to encourage discipline. Of course, the first thing you are going to do is keep playing ball, because if it is the first time, we tell you, you will try how far we get.

Once he did it to challenge us or frankly, he throws to break something, what we do is take the ball away. As we are not going to remove it forever, whenever we set the limit, we must give it a term. Thus, we will promote discipline in children.

Tips to educate children in self-discipline:

1. ***Remember that setting appropriate limits is not at odds with love.*** We must be firm before the norms that our children must meet for their good and the good of others, but to impose them with understanding and love.

2. ***Set limits without explaining why it can lead to manifest rebellion in adolescence.*** At these ages, they will shut up, but then they will rebel. Therefore, whenever I tell you why you can't do that, you must explain it to him until he assumes it.

3. ***When our children make us too nervous, and we no longer know what to do ("I told you an hour ago that you keep your clothes"), remember that physical punishment never educates. It merely relieves tension.*** If we observe that we want to give him a cake, we should force him to lock himself in his room and wait for both of you and him to be more relaxed.

4. ***Disrespect and answers are some of the limits you should always put.*** It is not that you do not stand that contradicts you. It is about internalizing that he should address you with education and respect, which is a consequence of love. And talk to your child about this matter, and if he does not comply, he should retire to his room and not leave it until he can apologize and speak respectfully to the same audience (siblings, older people) to which you disrespected. Afterward, you can discuss your differences.

Discipline in education.

One component of being a good father or mother is instilling discipline in our children. The discipline is a necessary part of childhood because it teaches children important concepts such as authority, abides by the rules, self-control, and responsibility. The discipline does not have to subtract spontaneity, happiness, and joy to our children. Instead, it gives them the freedom to explore and experience life within the safe limits that we have set for them.

All children, intrinsically, are born with a series of desires and preferences. From the first moments of life, we see how our children already begin to manifest their innate characteristics. Herein lies the beauty of individuality. However, our little ones do not know what is good or bad for them. They do not have the necessary experiences, they cannot foresee the consequences of their actions, and they have no way of controlling their desires and their impulses if we do not teach them how to do it.

The discipline is simply a way to show our children how we want to behave so that they are well, and nothing happens to them, so they are well-fed, physically active and healthy, and to become excellent and friendly people. We teach you these life lessons to help you integrate seamlessly into all types of groups, at school, and in your social environment.

Four effective tips.

A few guiding principles are all you need to instill your child discipline safely and effectively:

1. ***Set limits and stick to them.*** Children are only able to assimilate boundaries and boundaries if we, as parents, have them systematically respected. Children learn better and faster if we always apply the same limits and the same behavioral expectations. It is not efficient to create rules for when we are away from home if they are not also respected at home.

Example: If we want our son to sit at the table correctly, eat with the fork and speak quietly and without shouting when he is at the table, we have to practice and encourage these behaviors at home and systematically, so that when we go to eat outside know how to behave as expected of them.

2. ***Limits cannot be negotiated with the child.*** Our son does not know what is best for him. Our desires are free desires, which can be the result of many different motivations. It is not they who have to choose their limits. We, as parents, know what is best for them. That our children live up to our expectations is our responsibility. Children can try to oppose, but we have to help them follow our instructions to the end and in the way we choose, not them. It is essential that we, as parents, we are, maintain power and authority.

Example: If we want our children to turn off the television and go to bed when we tell them it is time to go to sleep, we cannot say "Yes" when they ask us to stay "5 more minutes".

3. ***Teach him what rights and obligations are.*** Everyone is born with rights and obligations. When we live in a community, as is the case with a family, each member has a series of rights and responsibilities that must be fulfilled so that everything works like silk. Teaching children from an early age, what rights and obligations are helping them understand that following a series of rules (requirements) allows them to access their rights.

Example. A 4-year-old girl does not want to put her shoes on; she wants mom to put them on. Mom has told him that if she wants to go to the park, she has to put on her shoes alone, like an older girl. Mom gives her daughter 5 minutes to put on her shoes. If you put on your shoes before the end of the 5 minutes, you will go to the park. If not, Mom will explain that they no longer have time to go to the park to play because they have wasted all the time waiting for her to finish putting on her shoes. Mom mustn't extend the agreed time to put on her shoes, or she will lose her authority with that gesture.

4. ***Maintain discipline as a discipline.*** It is helpful for parents to make it clear that discipline is something that is in effect, and that is being applied in the family. It is essential that the child does not feel confused or have doubts about the intentions or motivations of the parents in this regard. When a child does something that needs to be corrected, the parents should immediately show a bright and precise change of attitude to capture the child's attention and make them see that discipline is being put into practice.

Typically, this change in attitude includes the following elements: use the child's name when we talk to him, direct eye contact, a lower than normal voice, serious face, and a clear and sincere conversation (using tone and vocabulary appropriate to its degree of maturity) in which you explain what you have done wrong and how it should be corrected. After that, the father or mother must return to his usual attitude to show that the "moment of teaching" is over.

Using jokes or sarcasm can confuse children. Also, the help of rhetorical questions can be equally confusing and unclear. Children may not be able to know when parents are imposing discipline and when they are in a funny plan. Defining a clear standard of discipline helps a lot to clarify the situation and avoid ambiguities.

Example. Juan knows he can't play ball inside the house. Juan ignores this simple rule and unintentionally hits a painting on the wall, and that falls to the ground. The father listens to the noise and calls Juan by name. When Juan arrives where his father is, he says in a low voice and with a severe face, "You knew that in our family one of the rules is that you cannot play ball at home. You have not obeyed that rule and, because of it, you've broken a painting. You are grounded this weekend and, also, you will have to do some more homework than usual. Go and pick up the broken frame. We will talk later about the extra chores you'll have to do." Later, Juan and his father talk about the importance of family rules and norms.

For some parents, discipline may seem like a hard and arduous issue, but when discipline is applied based on love and affection, it becomes a tool for raising happy and self-confident children. All of us are subject to some discipline in our lives, the police in our city, our boss at work, or regulatory agencies (e.g., Treasury) at the state level. Children need to learn this discipline from their parents to be able to implement self-control, which will make them confident and capable of facing their mistakes or problems without undermining their self-esteem.

CHAPTER ELEVEN

Characteristics of A Bad Application Of The Discipline Or Errors.

Perhaps we will ask ourselves why to address the issue of mistakes or the wrong application of the discipline because, in my opinion, it is essential since as it is said "From mistakes you learn," or on many occasions we do not we realize them and repeat them regularly, this does not mean that we are bad parents or bad educators, what it tells us is that we can improve, it is also appropriate to mention that throughout this writing not only the errors will be mentioned but also aspects of how we can achieve effective discipline.

Parents and educators can adopt defined styles of education, and that in many cases are not the best, which can have consequences in the child, since many times methods are used that are at the extremes and do not reach a midpoint, there are a series of ways that do not give effective results, which are:

- ***Rigid Methods:***

Through this the figures of authority parents or teachers have all the power and the rules, that is they are too strict, consequences are not administered, but punishments, the needs of the child or opinions are not taken into account, in this model adults are right, and there is no discussion since the child is only trained to follow instructions, obey and perhaps the child behaves "well," can be given security, stability, and predictability, which can be considered as advantages, however, what is achieved when they grow up is that they are children without initiative, little capacity to make decisions, little creativity. Also, that responsibility is not encouraged, these children may become rebellious, have poor self-esteem, or be dependent on the opinions of other people.

- ***Permissive methods***:

This method is opposite to the previous one, the expression is given way, the creativity develops, the feelings, opinions, ideas of the child are taken into account, and the opportunity is given to make the decisions, about whether or not they do homework, if they want to help in the housework or not, etc., That is, few or no rules are established, they also do not administer consequences because it is believed that the child will learn from experience, however in this method it is not taken keep in mind that the child cannot self-regulate their behaviors and make long-term decisions, this can generate anxiety, insecurity, reduced capacity to meet their needs and do not recognize the importance of things, often these children grow up and fail to adapt to social norms and are frustrated by the lack of tools to face life, since with this type of education no skills are created, and children lack structure to achieve goals.

- ***Combination of methods:***

Many parents want to find the midpoint and seek to move from rigid discipline to permissive, and vice versa, when stiffness does not work they pass to permissiveness and do so indiscriminately, which causes insecurity, inconsistencies, extreme contradictions in the child and the child does not He manages to understand how he should act or not act, because at times we want the child to respect our authority, and at other times we allow him to do what he wants.

Methods used by our parents.

Sometimes parents, as they do not know how to handle their children, decide to take the pattern that their parents used with them. However, we were part of that discipline, and many times what our parents did was not pleasant for us. Now it is essential to understand that the generations are different, and each child is different, so what we learned as children may not apply to our children.

Copy some methods used by another person.

Sometimes we do not know how to react and instead try a method used by another person that has worked. Just because it worked for someone else does not mean it'll work for you or your child.

Errors That Parents Commit Frequently.

As we can see, there are various ways or methods of educating that are inappropriate for children, in addition to many of our behaviors as educators or parents do not cause a proper development of the child or on the contrary, they cause damage, so I will mention some mistakes that we can make discipline children, in which we can work to improve as parents or educators.

Reacting based on impulses and emotions can be shared in educators. Act without thinking, and you can hit or harm a child, not only physically but also emotionally, since it is only about resolving the conflict that you have at the moment, without reflecting and realizing what happens, in what circumstances is happening and how I can face it so that it is not recurrent.

The strategies we use with children are sometimes excellent. However, there is no time for them to give results, and it is continually changing to get what we are looking for quickly. The solutions are not always immediate. We must provide every effort sufficient time to work. For example, if a child does not like to do homework, and we make him see that it is his responsibility to do it, and he does not fulfill it, he will not be able to do any of his favorite activities like watching television. This is usually a good strategy, but many times it doesn't work because we expect the child to learn and do his homework for the first time, and he doesn't need us to be consistent and constant.

Many times we don't know how to react to the behaviors or attitudes of children, which causes them to be undecided, and this is usually a mistake since children perceive it. This affects their feelings of safety and well-being. Being indecisive can allow the child to be careless and dominant, which provides the child with the chance to do what he wants, without respecting rules and regulations.

There are many behaviors or behaviors that we want to change in children. However, we do not analyze the causes or nature of the actions that we want to change. This is why our change strategies do not work. It is necessary to investigate why this behavior arises, and from there, we will find a way to solve it. For example, if a child throws a tantrum over not getting candy at the store, what we do is buy the candy to avoid tantrum or crying. We do not realize that the outburst will occur every time the child wants candy since this gets results. On the contrary, what we must do is teach the child that the desired object can be obtained without tantrums, and sometimes it is not possible to buy the candy or get what he wants.

For convenience, laziness, lack of self-discipline, or simply because they learned it from their parents, children follow the teaching pattern and do not want to change. This is usually a grave mistake because all children are different. In addition to the natural development of the child, these teaching patterns lead us to the need to change these behavior patterns, which we find challenging. We prefer to continue despite not being the most convenient for them. It is what I know and has helped me achieve what I have so far, but it is essential to realize that the important thing is to adapt to their needs and characteristics.

Although as educators we believe that we have the control of the little ones in that we allow parents to manipulate their children, often without realizing it, through whims or making them feel guilty to authority figures with phrases such as "you are wrong, I hate you, I do not love you," etc. This makes us feel guilty, and we change it. This makes the child get to do what he wants. The child does not do it with the premeditation of "I am going to manipulate my parents," it is merely a means to get what he is looking for and he can do it if we allow him to feel guilty.

Some educators, mainly the parents, think that while the child is small, "you have to save him work because he will have to fight later." Activities or tasks are done for the children, or he is not allowed to help us in the work because the child does not perform the activities as we would like. Sometimes it takes us longer than if we do it for ourselves, and this is a huge mistake since the child is not allowed to learn to persevere and be responsible. What is achieved with these attitudes is that they are lazy. We spend time wanting to rest and killing time on things that will not be useful, or on the other hand, it is demanded of more, the children must carry out activities according to their age and their real capacities. If it is not so, the child will always be frustrated by not being able to perform the entrusted activities, which will generate him insecurity and anguish. It is, therefore, essential to know the characteristics of children and to know at least in a general way of child development.

On many occasions, there is a lack of agreement between parents when implementing discipline. What this achieves is that the child can manipulate the parents through tantrums. Sometimes the children give each parent a good or bad role, and this allows the children to have a figure that causes fear and another that is not taken as authority. The important thing is that the people in charge of the child reach an agreement on how to implement rules. If the parents don't agree, he can manipulate the parents to disagree and get what he wants, which gives him an excessive power to make decisions. This gives him an unreal feeling of authority, and the absence of effective control generates anxiety.

We may have a misconception of what love is for children. Many times we do not let them do anything for fear of what may happen to them. We do not allow them to be bothered, we do not let them take risks that are sometimes necessary for their development, and we would like to keep the child in a glass bubble. We consent too much, and we may mistakenly believe that what we are doing is the best. However, there is overprotection, and instead of showing the child how much we love him, we create an insecure, shy, indecisive creature, accustomed to others acting and deciding instead.

Introducing fears is to disarm and limit the child. It is essential to realize that fear disorganizes and weakens the mind, inhibits it, creates shyness, and also damages the psyche. Many times we as educators are afraid of something and transmit the fear to children. If we teach him to fear something new, we can help increase or decrease the anxiety. If we are altered, we cause the child to improve his fear, and if we are calm and give him security, this fear will diminish little by little.

On the other hand, fear is also instilled in the child to gain control over them. Many times the child is told: "if you misbehave, the devil takes you," which does not lead the child to learn something productive. They are harmed, and this is often done by not hitting or scolding them, and we believe it is the best solution, but it is necessary to reconsider and find other ways to maintain control of the children.

The boredom of the students: some students seem to have no discipline problems although they are tremendously bored. However, they have developed "adaptation" strategies. Not all have been able to create them and do not hide their boredom despite the consequences that their behavior generates. In these cases, a discipline problem occurs where both the teacher and the student are responsible.

Another mistake that I think is very important to mention is that the dignity of the child is often compromised. The pride not only does not physically assault since the child is also attacked with a phrase such as "You are a fool," "I can't stand you," "I am fed up," and "You never do things right," which makes the child internalize the ideas and come to believe them. This causes an effect on the self-concept of the child that is negative and gives him insecurities.

The aggressions, both physical and verbal, we believe many times that can help us control the child and make them do what we expect. However this attacks the child in his bodily, psychological, emotional integrity and perhaps he will be able to perform what you want, however, is how he will learn to get others to do what he wants through aggressions to others weaker than him, and they are patterns that are repeated throughout the generations.

We can use guilt to make the child feel responsible for everything wrong that happens, and his presence is considered the discomfort of others. He is prepared to believe that he is terrible and does not have many alternatives to change according to the vision of adults. This makes the child insecure and fearful, with a poor self-concept, with this I do not mean that he is not responsible for his actions but not to leave all responsibility to him and make him see how he can change his actions.

Due to the hectic world that we live in, many times, the child puts at an emotional distance, which causes him to feel a lack of affection. He already needs physical or emotional contact, and this can cause him to perceive that we do not want it from him or that there is something wrong with it. This can influence their future relationships with other people. Another essential aspect that can harm them is rejection, whether it is said explicitly or implicitly. This affects the child's safety and causes low self-esteem.

Adults sometimes want the child to be still, not play and not touch; it is necessary to understand that he plays and has a lot of activity. This is his way of knowing the world. Preventing him from playing and moving implies that he does not learn and delay his development, of course, this must-have limits and control; It is a mistake to believe that the success of an appropriate discipline is measured by obedience, but by many other aspects such as the self-control that the child has and the values that he demonstrates day by day.

Children, according to the complaints of some parents are disobedient, but many times the mistake is that we give absurd or ambiguous orders or instructions, that the child cannot understand or fulfill, we only tell him what we do not want him to do, but we do not give alternatives of what to do.

Before concluding, I think it is essential to recognize one of the biggest mistakes that "ignorance" can make; that is, there is no general culture. There is a lack of physiological and psychological information about childhood; this can cause many problems regarding the discipline of our children.

The above are mistakes that as educators, parents, teachers, and people close to children we make, often without realizing it. The important thing is not to blame someone or worry that we are not doing the right thing, but in my view, it is essential to recognize that we have what we do is not the most convenient and look for ways to improve.

To conclude this chapter, it is necessary to recognize that each of these mentioned errors is feasible to be corrected by ourselves and avoid them as much as possible. However, it is essential to put considerable effort into knowing how we can help the little ones and put that knowledge into practice.

CHAPTER TWELVE

How to put your newborn on a schedule.

Caring for a child is difficult but getting your baby ready to sleep and eat on a regular schedule can help make things easier. Most experts agree an infant is likely to have a routine between the ages of two and four months.

1. **Establish a daytime schedule.**

Make notes about the routine for your child. It is recommended that you buy a notebook before you start, in which you keep a record of your baby's daily schedule. This will help identify whether the new plan works.

- Create a simple table with the following columns on the first page of the notebook: time, activity, notes. Take note of every significant incident that happens throughout the day, every weekday. Write, for instance, "6 a.m.: the baby wakes up, 9 a.m.: the baby eats, 11 a.m.: the baby takes a nap, etc."

- Similarly, you can keep track of your baby's schedule in an inventory on your computer or use an online registration service such as Trixie Tracker or Baby Insights.

Create a schedule based on your baby's natural rhythm. Try to look out if there is any regularity in the current cycle of feeding and resting your baby.

- You can try to incorporate diaper changes and your baby's moodiness into your schedule if you notice that he tends to need a diaper change or if he is moody at a time of day.

- This will make it easier to adapt to your new schedule and help you plan your day based on your baby's needs.

- A baby who is not deprived of sleep or who is not hungry will be happier and more willing to play, snuggle, and learn new things.

The first thing you should do is set a time to wake up. Although it can be difficult, you will have to wake up your baby at the same time every day, even if he is sleeping. You will have to adapt the baby's nap schedule so that he sleeps later if he tends to wake up before the time you want him to wake up.

Try to set a standard time to wake up. Newborns usually sleep a lot during the day. During the first weeks, they need sixteen hours of sleep a day.

- Because sleep is a primary activity for infants, it is necessary to give some order in that activity to prevent them from waking up in the middle of the night.

Feed your baby, change it, and play with it. When the baby wakes up, change his diaper, and dress him for the day. Then, hold your baby close to you and let her feed. No matter if you feed your baby with breast milk or baby milk powder, he needs to feel close to you.

- Play with your baby after feeding him. Talk to him, sing to him and snuggle with him. He will like your smell, your voice, and your closeness.

- After playing, lay the baby down for a nap. Do it as soon as you notice signs of fatigue, such as yawning, irritability, crying, or movements to touch your nose.

Let the baby sleep for two or three hours. The baby will probably wake up after two or three hours. If he doesn't, you should wake him up. A baby who sleeps too much will not eat enough during the day and can become dehydrated and lose weight.

Repeat this cycle in the day. You can repeat the cycle mentioned earlier in the day, except it is advised that you feed the baby before you change the diaper and play. This is because many babies use their diapers while they eat. This way, you will avoid changing it twice. Therefore, do the following:

- Wake the baby to take a nap.

- Feed the baby.

- Change your baby's diapers, then play with him for a moment, talk, sing, and snuggle.

- Make the baby fall asleep again.

Make a difference between sleeping day and night. To establish a sleep schedule for your baby at night, you must make a distinction between sleeping at night and during the day.

- You can do this by letting the baby sleep in a room with daylight and a dark room at night. Putting the baby to take a nap in a dark room will only confuse him and ruin his sleep pattern.

- Do not be afraid to make noise when the baby takes a nap in the day as he needs to learn to get used to it. Leave the radio on, use the vacuum cleaner, and speak with a reasonable volume.

Feed your baby when he is hungry. You must notice that you should always feed the baby when he is hungry, even if that does not fit your schedule.

- It's not fair for a newborn to go hungry just because feeding him doesn't fit your schedule.

- The signs that your baby is hungry are crying, and he sucks his hand.

Feed your baby every two to three hours when you feed him with breast milk. You should feed your baby every two to three hours, even if she doesn't cry or doesn't seem to want to eat. This is very important when breastfeeding with breast milk.

- The mother's breasts can be congested with milk if the baby does not eat at this rate, which can be painful for the mother and what could make it difficult to feed the baby.

- The mother's breasts will not have time to accumulate enough milk, and the quality and quantity of the milk will decrease if the baby is fed very frequently. In this case, the baby may be starving, even though he eats continuously.

2. **Set a night schedule.**

Set a time to sleep. Look at the baby's natural time and find out the best time for her to go to bed. Having a diary will be useful for this.

- Do not play too much with the newborn before bedtime. It can be very stimulating, which makes it more difficult for you to sleep.

- Bath the baby before bedtime and massage his skin with milk or baby oil. This will relax you before bedtime.

At night, reduce noise levels. Sing your baby a lullaby or play a piece of soft and silent music to sleep. Sing even if you are not skilled at it. Your baby loves your voice and is not a music critic.

- Make almost no noise in the house during the night. A quiet and peaceful environment will indicate to your baby that it is not a regular nap.

Reduce the light. Put your baby to sleep in a room with low light. Don't turn on the lights completely; you always must be able to see your baby. The dark environment will help you sleep at night.

Get ready for your baby to wake up during the night. The baby is likely to wake up during the night. When this happens, take it in your arms, feed it and put it to sleep. Do not change your diaper unless it is essential. That part is omitted from the nighttime, in addition to games and snuggling.

- Wake the baby if he does not wake up during the night to eat. No matter how good it may sound to let a newborn sleep through the night, it is not healthy for him.

- Babies must eat every two to three hours. Otherwise, the baby may become dehydrated and hungry, causing fatigue and weakness.

Respect the baby's schedule as much as possible. It is essential to do so, especially the times for sleeping and waking up. This way, it will be easier for your baby to get used to it. However, keep in mind that over time, your baby will sleep less and require more of your attention and time.

CHAPTER THIRTEEN

Values That We Have to Teach Children.

Childhood is the most precious moment of any person, and it is also the stage in which we learn. It is when we begin to form our concepts and models. Your son will learn from you, and he will feed on you. You are his mother and his first and most precious role model. That is why you should try to stay close to good, beauty, loyalty, truth, and love because these are the five values that we have to teach children.

It is in our childhood when we learn to recognize what is good and what is bad, what makes us good, what makes us courageous, what makes us advance. That is the stage in which we recognize the dangers that could damage our body and our life. We learn that fire can burn us, that electricity can harm us if we do not use it properly and understand that being careful keeps us from physical and emotional pain.

When we are children, we try, like every living being, to be close to what makes us good, healthy, and comfortable. The most significant amount of well-being and security comes from our Mom; that's why we want to be always close to her and her heart.

On the other hand, you, as a mother, have the privilege, the happiness, and the responsibility of having the children of your children in your hands. The task of teaching should be subtle and sweet, qualities that feed primarily on a relationship based on solidarity and love.

The first thing that moms should teach their children is to appreciate how valuable they are and all the possibilities he has at his fingertips just by merely being alive. On this basis, your child will learn what is right for him and will also do well. You will appreciate the good as a value.

The value of good.

Ensuring the welfare of a person as unique as a child involves so much effort and, at the same time, requires so much love that only a mother can accomplish such a commendable task. Ensuring the good of a child means making sure that he is fed, that his body and his environment are clean, that he maintains his good health, and that his basic needs are satisfied so that he can continue to grow.

All mothers instinctively ensure the well-being of their child, it is written in their genetic code, and their first mission is to preserve the life of their child, who is undoubtedly the most beautiful and delicate creature they have ever seen—his eyes.

But beyond the basic needs, every mother must ensure the emotional well-being of her beloved son, and she does it every day, with her best and highest effort, providing security, tranquility, peace, peace.

In doing so, the child is learning that he must behave in a way that preserves his physical integrity, his health, and his emotional well-being. The child who knows how to distinguish what is good for him, what is good for him, and humanity in general, will do all those things that do him good.

That child who does good will be an adult who will eat healthily, who will sleep for the hours he needs, who will surround himself with people who value him and help him grow, who will know how to identify and take care of everything good for him.

The value of beauty.

When you think of beauty, the image of a landscape, a flower, or the stars inevitably comes to mind. Beauty, although it could also be associated with the image of a supermodel, can be seen in its maximum splendor in nature, in the creatures and phenomena that exist on planet earth and in the universe, among which are human beings.

Most people admire beauty, and surely you are among them. If you unravel what you like about it, you will discover that you like order, softness, luminosity, freshness. All these aspects can be achieved by admiring the beauty of a landscape or the face of a person. You can also find them inside each human being, a soul that exudes beauty for the coherence of its acts and thoughts, for the order it carries in its life, for the smoothness with which it is conducted, for the luminosity it gives off.

Most human beings are looking for beauty. Identifying it, valuing it, and cultivating it is an art that your child will surely be able to master as he seeks his inner beauty.

Loyalty, one of the values you should teach your child.

The education of your children consists in filling their possibilities with strength, giving security to their wishes, accepting their decisions, and teaching them to be true to themselves. One of the greatest satisfactions of life is to follow the opinion of your heart, be faithful to your essence, your principles, your dreams, and achieve your goals.

Your child may change his mind and not study medicine, for example. What you do will not be too decisive if you are following his heart, teach him to listen, to have loyalty with his values, with his principles, that will give you the peace of mind that a good heart always guides his determinations.

The value of the true.

You will have already experienced that this world is full of much falsehood, of many objects that sell as jewels, but that is a fantasy that eventually turns black. That sense of falsehood is sometimes also found in the feelings of some people, in whom we hoped to find true love, true friendship, true loyalty, but, instead, we found falsehood and oops! How it hurts to find fantasy where we hoped to find gold.

So, to teach your child to recognize the truth and give it courage, as a mother, you must exercise in understanding and valuing it. You already know what some of the signs of truth are; For example, a piece of gold, like a real friendship, does not deteriorate, does not blacken over time. Time does not harm the truth. It transforms it, it models it, but it does not hurt it.

And so, little by little, with attention to detail, you will learn to decipher what is right and what is not. Many adults already know it; mothers especially know about true love; they experience it daily with their children whom they must teach to identify the truth, the truth, and appreciate it as the great treasure that it is.

The value of love.

You are the one who takes care of your child's future, giving shelter, care, fun, time for the game, security, peace, solidarity, are just some signs of love. You, as a mother, now know more than ever what love all is about, you know that loving is an unconditional act that is not affected by external agents.

Now that you learn with your son to love, he also learns with you; he is your teacher and your disciple. Both will learn that when you love a flower, you love all flowers, that when you love yourself honestly, time does not wreak havoc, neither does distance or even what the other person does, love is unconditional.

When you love your child, he learns to recognize love, to identify it, to practice it, to receive it, and to give it. Love is the only thing we live for, it is what makes us free, what makes us feel alive.

CHAPTER FOURTEEN

The 7 Foods You Should Never Give Your Baby.

In the first four months of life, the baby must maintain his exclusive diet through breastfeeding. In some cases, the baby needs to be given some milk formula, but the food par excellence in the first stage of his life is breast milk.

However, after the four months have passed, an adaptation period begins in which the child can receive additional feeding, which serves as a complement to breastfeeding. These foods are usually simple and light, which is generally very similar in all families.

Mothers began to supplement the baby's diet with soft, natural, and simple porridge. The fruit porridge is typical in the snack, then other products that are not of the dairy family are gradually incorporated.

Therefore, you must be cautious so that new foods are not harmful to your small organism. It is also necessary to adapt the preparation and the quantity of the product, to facilitate its digestion and promote its maturation.

Seven foods you should never feed your baby.

Although sometimes it is inevitable that children eat certain foods, with babies it should be less complicated because mothers are responsible for the preparation of their meals and as babies should not consume more than their milk or some natural porridge.

However, sometimes due to ignorance or lack of interest, we fall into unhealthy eating routines for the little ones. In this sense, although it is not a custom, there are some foods that babies should not consume for any reason.

Even if it does not seem like it, certain foods are preferable that are not part of the diet of children under 12 months and only in moderation from that age, up to four years. Not everyone knows what they are, but there are also cases in which we ignore the advice of the pediatrician.

To take care of the health of our children, we must remember that these seven products must be eliminated from the usual food we administer at home. These might be:

1. The Sugar.

This food, although very common, does not need the baby because breast milk contains it. If our idea is to sweeten the food to improve its flavor, we can do it through fruits. Also, sugar can cause premature tooth decay.

2. Honey.

It is a natural substitute for sugar, whose use in the feeding of children is very recurrent; But what we don't know is that its composition is very similar to that of white sugar. Another drawback is the possibility that it contains dangerous bacteria for the digestive system.

3.The Salt.

Like honey and sugar, salt is used to highlight the taste of food. It is also harmful. This product should be removed from the diet of infants because it threatens the health of the kidneys. It is only recommended moderately after twelve months.

4. Marine species.

Certain types of fish and shellfish possess high amounts of mercury, an element that is a product of pollution. Therefore, it is present in all oceans. This makes it possible for fish to consume and accumulate in their body.

5. Some vegetables.

Algae, chard, spinach, and borage, whose composition contains nitrate; in excessive amounts, they could cause the decrease of oxygen in the blood. This as a result of its transformation to nitrites.

Although we talk about excessive consumption, it is contraindicated in babies because their body is small and therefore of higher concentration.

6. Low fat modified products.

It is not wrong to consume products with less fat, but we are talking about those skimmed ones, which have undergone special procedures to eliminate excess fat. On the other hand, the fats of these foods are essential for the organism of the small ones, are a source of vitamins and calories.

7. Some foods according to your presentation.

Food can be consumed in different preparations or presentations, which can modify its properties considerably. That is why you should avoid feeding the baby, not quite the food, but the way it is administered.

Therefore, it is necessary to avoid raw preparations of animal origin, nuts without crushing, drinks based on rice, French fries, meringues, ice cream, among others.

CHAPTER FIFTEEN

Baby Temperament and Personality Can Affect Baby's Sleep.

Personality is described as how a child responds naturally to circumstances and stimuli, its mood, its ability to control itself, and its level of activity. Most researchers believe that personality is innate, which means that this is how a child is programmed to be and is not a product of its climate.

The personality of a baby may influence which method of sleep training a parent may choose to help her baby sleep better. The temperament and character of a child will decide whether a no-cry sleep training system takes one hour or three months, or whether he is more likely to cry for five minutes or two hours if he prefers a scream-method.

The way a baby reacts to being wet, hungry, or tired may not be like a neighbor's baby from the first day after they're born. Where one baby may be low-key and not very distressed, another baby can loudly cry out. This is also the reason why one method of sleep training works well for some babies and won't work for others.

Below are listed three common types of temperament and personality with a brief synopsis of how they may affect a baby's sleep.

Intensity:

The sensitivity of a baby or toddler is how strongly she responds emotionally to something. This could be in a good or bad manner. Since babies with high intensity react strongly, it means they may squeal loudly with excitement or cry aloud because they are wet. For babies with low intensity, this can mean that when they are uncomfortable, they hardly ever cry or fuss.

How could the pressure of a baby affect its sleep? If a child is a baby with low intensity, this means that putting the baby down drowsy may be much more comfortable but wake up from a very early age and help her learn to sleep alone.

If your baby is a baby of high intensity, it will be difficult to leave her frustrated when she is young for anything more than a few minutes. A baby with high intensity may get more upset when she wakes up between cycles of sleep and cannot go back to sleep. It may also take longer to soothe a high-intensity baby before sleep during the bedtime routine. If you're trying to use a no-cry sleep training method, likely, a high-intensity baby will still weep, and it can be tough to listen to a screaming baby while trying to break sleep associations, and it will be much harder to stick to when she gets upset. If you use a form of weeping sleep training, expect loud and long outbursts and shouts.

Persistence:

The strength of a baby is how easy or difficult it can halt a job if it is told and how strong-willed it is when it has its mindset on something. Persistence will show itself when a baby wants to nurse, and without erupting in tears, he won't take no for an answer and won't settle down with any other relieving process.

How could the persistence of a baby affect its sleep? If a child is a less stubborn infant, this means that getting better sleep out of her probably won't be difficult. Usually, babies and toddlers who are less stubborn take no for an answer and do not remain unhappy for very long when there are adjustments. Most parents need to commit to making changes to change the baby's sleep.

If a baby is very persistent, and he has his mind set on something, it will be harder to get more cooperation out of him. If you use a form of no-cry sleep training, it will probably take longer than those with less frequent children. Sadly, if you want to use a crying sleep training process, expect long bouts of crying. This may or may not be challenging to get through, depending on his level of intensity.

Perceptiveness:

The perceptiveness of a baby is how much an infant senses such things as objects, colors, and noises. A perceptive child can forget directions or instructions given to her because her attention has been drawn to something else. She might also notice other things other people may not be able to do, like a rock in the grass that other children might walk past. Perceptivity and distinctiveness are not the same as ADHD.

How could the perceptiveness of a baby affect his or her sleep? The perceptiveness of your child will most affect sleep when it comes to napping, habits night light can also have more effect on their sleep in a perceptive child's room than less observant children would. When doing the bedtime routine, a toddler may not be able to follow multi-step instructions, and thus benefit from breaking down the habits into smaller steps.

It may take her longer to fall asleep than a child who isn't as alert simply because she sees more in the house. For this reason, it will be necessary to put a more alert baby down of bed at least 10-15 minutes early to allow them time to relax.

Knowing that a parent can learn and understand the temperament of their child and be able to predict how they will react to certain things is essential. People who recognize the personality of their baby or child will help support the child in ways that make their disposition fit well with that. Once parents know the temperament of their baby, it can help to reduce some of the stress associated with supporting their baby learn to sleep better as they will not always try to figure out why he is reacting in a certain way.

Even though the temperament of a child is biological, this does not mean that it does not matter what the parents do. Parents will be able to show the strengths of their children, help them understand their personality, and help them learn how to deal with their reactions as they grow up. It's not only challenging to try to make him forget his temperamental tendencies, but it's also telling him not to be himself.

While many assume like sleep deprivation is the only alternative, or crying it out, there is a range of other options to put a baby to sleep. Understanding the personality of a baby can help to determine the approach best suited to teaching healthy sleep patterns to an infant.

Baby Sleeping Tips.

Baby sleeping problems and issues have become a concern for many parents because of the different children's sleep patterns. You'll find very few parents content with their babies ' sleep amount or sleep patterns. Some parents complain that the baby is not sleeping well, or that their timing for sleep is not normal. The parents are also expected to have disturbed sleep unless the baby sleeps soundly, which makes life very difficult for them.

Because of many different reasons, a baby may have a problem sleeping soundly. Therefore, parents must first identify the causative factor before the issue of sleep can be solved. The baby may be reluctant to sleep because it is hungry, or because the baby bedding on which the baby is made to sleep is not comfortable or cozy. Yes, one of the most common factors contributing to baby sleep disruptions is the bedding of poor quality. It is often seen that the baby wants to sleep on the lap of his mother, instead of the crib set for baby bedding.

Here are some useful ideas that will help you overcome baby sleep disorders:

The distinction between night and daytime should be explained to the children. If they are trained to differentiate between day and night. They will soon realize when it's time to sleep and when they're supposed to play. It means setting the babies a sleeping schedule-you need to give the babies a regular bedtime routine, which will allow them to have a good nighttime sleep. The incremental improvement of consistent sleep timing would undoubtedly help to reduce infant sleep disorders.

Discomfort in bedtime is another explanation for babies not willing to sleep. You must ensure the baby's baby bedding or baby bedding crib set is safe. They may be reluctant to sleep if they are uncomfortable in their baby bedding or the baby bedding crib set. Therefore, you can check to see if the baby bedding or the baby bedding crib set is put in a comfortable place, without noises or noisy sounds to scare off the child. If the crib set is put in an unventilated environment, the baby can find it very uncomfortable.

You must ensure the baby's room is clean and airy. The room temperature should be reasonably comfortable-neither too cold nor too dry.

Check to ensure that the blankets provided with bassinet baby bedding are not very tightly wrapped around the baby's body and provide enough space for the baby to sleep comfortably. The baby's clothes should also be checked, and should they be loosened to allow the baby to sleep comfortably in case they are too tight.

Another exciting factor that can ensure your baby is sleeping well is related to their hunger patterns. Many moms fail to understand that the baby is hungry because he doesn't want to sleep. So, you need to make sure your baby isn't hungry, and its tummy is full.

You should take the little one in your arms and keep it tight to your body in case the baby starts to weep continuously in the baby bedding, or the baby bedding crib package. You can also gently rock the baby in your arms, or on a rocking chair. Rocking will make your baby happy and will make you sleep better.

Besides your baby bedding crib kit, you can also play soft music or gently sing a lullaby so that your baby sleeps off.

Baby Sleep Tips When Teething.

Many parents wonder if teething could affect their baby's sleep. The teething sometimes begins just after a baby starts to sleep through the night. This can be upsetting for many parents, especially for new parents, as they thought the whole tiring night had now come to an end, but it unexpectedly returned. It doesn't mean that everything your baby has accomplished with independent sleeping needs to go out of the window.

Teething will begin at age four to six months. It may take, however, sometime before the actual tooth emerges.

Teething may take up to two years of age and may contribute to the waking of the toddler night. Many babies have mild signs of teething like drooling and chewing on everything, while other babies may have severe symptoms of puffiness and crankiness as the tooth pops through. Thus, one baby differs from one baby to another that one may have a peaceful sleep, while others may have frequent waking during teething.

You may have heard that some experts say that teething won't interrupt baby's sleep, but each baby isn't the same as others and will have different tolerances of pain.

It would be your job as parents to understand how teething affects them, and to have sympathy for them. And don't forget to make sure they get enough sleep, too.

Two places are affected by its teething in your baby's sleep:

- Wakes early in the morning. Your baby can wake up earlier than average when teething and find it hard to get himself back to sleep.

- Hard to snuggle. Teething baby takes longer to fall asleep and a shorter nap at nap time. It is also possible he could skip the rest too. That can be up to a week for a few days. Just note it's temporary, so you don't have to put up with pain.

These are some things you need to take while coping with your baby's sleep problem when he is in the teething phase:

- As a baby's teething can take up to two years of age, and it can be both on and off, it would be best to have a strategy on how to handle the situation, which in this case is your loved one's sleeping problem. You need to remember not only one location in which your loved one is tired of having restless night as he is in distress but also yourself and another family member who can also have a disturbed night's sleep. The period will last from 2 to 4 days, and your baby will need extra shooting at these times until the tooth comes out of his gum.

- You can give him Motrin, or people always use Bonjela when you're in Australia, and those two are known to be quite reliable. Until giving your baby any drugs, however, please check the dose and another factor with your child's doctor first.

- Expect your baby will want to eat more if you breastfeed him, as it offers mental and gum support as well.

- At his teething period, you can still start your baby's sleep training. But in those 2-4 days of peak time maybe be a little bit gentle and accommodating to him.

Why Baby Sleep Is So Important.

Sleep - something we all need. It's important to parents, babies, children and well, everyone! Sadly, many of us don't get enough of it-including our children.

We all need sufficient amounts of sleep to function correctly, and these babies and young children need to develop. It is well known that adults with sleep deprivation have difficulties in focusing and operating and can suffer long-term mental and physical health problems. Often, when sleep is disrupted, one cannot expect an exhausted baby to function effectively either!

For physical and mental rejuvenation, a working immune system, healthy growth, and emotional well-being, sleep is essential. Your baby will become fretful, irritable, and inconsolable without enough sleep. And to make matters worse, early childhood sleep-deprivation will further mess with their potential for deep, restful sleep over the longer term.

Babies and children who do not get enough sleep are often unjustly branded as' fussy' and' temperamental' when they are too tired to function correctly. Babies suffering from this poor sleep quality often have parents who are also exhausted and thus unable to enjoy, care for, and nurture their children as they wish.

- More than 70 percent of infants and infants have some kind of sleep problem, according to a recent study by the National Sleep Association.

- About 50 percent of babies suffering from sleep issues will continue to experience problems through pre-school and school-age if not treated.

- Insufficient sleep is detrimental to health, actions, mood, attention, memory, and learning ability in babies and children.

Many parents think babies are irritable and inconsolable. "My child is crying all day even when he's awake...... of COURSE he's hard!" Fussy-yes. An irritable condition-no. Some babies maybe a little more sensitive and temperamental, but for some reason, babies who cry so much do. If there are no medical complications and a baby isn't in pain, then your baby can sleep during the day simply because he's tired! Even if he takes occasional cat naps here and there, the overall lack of sleep, which is so essential to his well-being, will not be solved.

Such first stuff. If you think your baby doesn't get enough sleep to work correctly and be well-rested, then it's time to do something about it. Take note of his daily behavior and ask yourself:

- How many naps does he take every day?

- How long do these naps last?

- How long will he stay awake between naps?

- How much sleep does he get in the evening?

After you have figured out the underlying patterns of your baby, you might want to reconfigure certain aspects of his daily sleep to ensure that your baby is well-rested and happy.

CHAPTER SIXTEEN

Survival Training Exercises with Babies and Children.

You cannot prepare properly when planning for an emergency survival situation if you leave half your family at home. You must take every member of the family with you when you have a survival exercise, or your time is nothing but wasted. Such family members should include babies and small children. Let's face it if these members are going to be with you in a real emergency, so don't leave them with a babysitter at home.

If you're fitted to stay in your vehicle, so half of your issues are over. But, if you need to use a tent of sorts, other additional considerations will have to be added because of the baby or the child. If preparing for your survival equipment as well as your methods, the safety and security of these little children should be foremost in your mind.

If you use a tent, you should find a smaller shelter as the baby's frame. This small enclosure, with its associated infant seat, will hold one baby. This enclosure is a screen enclosure that you place inside your tent to protect the baby from insects. This device prevents the baby from having bites from spiders and mosquitoes. Make sure to bring your baby a tiny sleeping bag that will be used inside your tent when the infant is not in the enclosure. This baby will feel much more secure when wrapped in a blanket in the sleeping bag.

The goal here is to make the baby feel more at ease and less apprehensive as he is not with his usual surroundings in his typical home. Until moving on your survival exercise, let the baby nap at home in the sleeping bag for a couple of nights to get him accustomed. Be sure you're making the baby's activity area to include his favorite toys or anything he's used to playing at home.

Since you don't have all the stuff you would like at home, you might want to carry some things to make the baby a little more relaxed. You can consider the pool of a small child and include some if the child is of age where he can play games anyway.

Stress your young children that correctly following the rules is imperative. Nevertheless, during the exercise, failure to comply even with the simplest of guidelines could have severe effects if it were an actual emergency. Provide a whistle for each child to hang around its neck. Inform them that this is a vital tool to save lives and not a toy. Tell them, and make them understand that if an emergency happens, they should blow the whistle then and only then. Also, let them know they should not be wandering away from the main camp. There are certainly side trips and hikes out.

Furthermore, if you use a tent, it is important to stress to your children that no food of any kind should ever enter the tent. Our drills are mostly in the forests where wild animals are sure to be roaming around. No food should ever be allowed inside your tent, even for a few cookies. Also, if this exercise is in a region where there are no known bears, the law should be followed. You must note that it is likely that raccoons and small animals, as well as insects, can circumvent your site even in case you are vigilant regarding food rules.

Instruct your child that no wild animals should ever approach, feed or pet, no matter how cute they may seem. If your child is at an age in which they can understand, then let them know about the possibility of rabies and wildlife.

A wet survival training trip will undoubtedly be less than enjoyable for young children and babies. To tackle these circumstances, make sure you bring a solar-powered flashlight and radio, or as I have the wind-up models now. Let the children turn-in details about the weather station to find out if the storm is going by, or of a more lasting nature. Don't automatically assume we can go home as well since it's storming. In a real-life situation, that is not a clear choice. Just sit back and let go of the storm. The children especially enjoy talking, playing games, telling their favorite stories, or simply reading in the tent.

A reason exercising that is advantageous to children in terms of health and development:

- Children are less likely to get overweight, so their body fat will be better controlled. Obese children can increase their body weight and fat due to the hormonal effect of consuming it during exercise.

- Studies report exercise increases children's mood and attitude, reduces anxiety, and decreases depression. The sleep quality is also improved.

- Exercising improves the heart and lungs and the cardiovascular system. The heart achieves a higher "pump-activity" when improving the child's heart and lungs, promoting heart disease prevention. Participating in regular physical activity prevents or impedes the progression of many chronic illnesses (diabetes, heart disease, obesity, and hypertension) and promotes wellness.

- Exercising helps to develop essential communication skills like team sports involvement.

- Exercise helps develop motor coordination and many other performance skills.

- Exercise increases metabolism in the brain. Studies show that activity encourages better attendance at school and improves performance at the academic level. Active children can concentrate much more, even after a long school session ends. Research shows that healthy children have enhanced memory as a result of better brain functioning.

- Exercise helps the body's ability to combat illness. Children are less likely to get colds, allergies, and diseases.

- Fun and moderate exercise burns off excess harmful hormones and increases positive hormone release.

- Children who keep fit are more energized because of the desire to detoxify their bodies. Healthy children breathe better and sweat more that are great ways of detoxifying the body and helping to keep it "clean."

- Active children enhance the ability of their own body to absorb oxygen through aerobic exercise; more oxygen equates to more energy. This increase in blood flow promotes the movement of the body's metabolism by-products and toxins back from the cells to be recycled, eliminated, or used in other body parts.

- Regular physical activity helps keep healthy muscles, joints, and bones alive and grow.

- Children playing and practicing are more likely to continue to work as an adult.

CHAPTER SEVENTEEN

Ways to Sleep Better as A New Parent.

1. Set the Focus mood to where everything happens. Consider your bedroom a haven from the day you and your partner are only allowed to go for two things: sleep and sex!

In associating your bedroom with just those two things, at the end of the day, you will be able to focus on your tiredness and ease yourself into sleep mode.

The surrounding area should be both cool and quiet. Anything short, constant, and calm will help if you need a bit of sound. They should also be as devoid of electronics as possible. They've been shown to hurt your sleep as well as being a constant distraction at the end of the day.

2. Escape the Day You've managed to set up your child's strict bedtime routine, but you still have the stuff to do. It's time to focus your spotlight on yourself.

Set up your bed routine. Make sure that from the day on, you can wind down.

Try avoiding alcohol. You can feel that you are getting to bed quicker, but your overall sleep will suffer. Hold snacks light and minimize screen time. While you might need some escape, try reading, playing a game, or setting your next day to-dos.

3. It's not just the role of a mom to bear all the responsibility for a new baby. It defines a way of sharing the load. It includes feedings for overnight stay and bedtime duties.

Longer sleep will help you sleep better. So, if you can split the night into shifts by passing from side to side over the baby monitor, then you and your partner may be able to enjoy some extra hours that can do wonders!

4. Getting up physically and getting active is essential. While a child can wear you out, setting up an exercise routine is not necessarily the same as setting up.

The benefits of exercise are well known. But the focus areas are how it gives you strength in the daytime and makes you fall asleep more quickly at the end of the day.

There's nothing unique to it (weight training, cycling, etc.); any physical activity will improve. But what you want to prevent is raising the heart rate too close to bedtime. Though after a late-night run, you can feel exhausted, your body won't be ready to wind down.

5. Look for help While this might mean seeking advice from a doctor (which is a viable option), what we mean is finding sleep aids that work for you. Sound machines, eye masks, chamomile tea all can help make you sleep quickly.

CHAPTER EIGHTEEN

Phrases to End Your Children's Tantrums.

There is no more complex challenge for a father than to placate tantrums. However, ending tantrums is possible, as long as we act correctly as adults. Under no circumstances is it about shouting, insulting, humiliating, threatening, or punishing the child.

Once again, communication is everything in our lives and that of our children. The dialogue is what will help us overcome these crises. Moreover, over time, you will see how the conversation will provide your child with the necessary tools to express what he feels correct.

But what is the additional secret?

The final sentence of these dialogues is always the most important. Of course, you should use it only in case your child does not want to understand what, and you have tired of explaining and repeating again and again with infinite patience. Do you want to know what it is about? Find out below!

How to end the tantrums?

First, a detail that cannot be missed is knowing exactly what a tantrum or tantrum is. Well, it is nothing more or nothing less than the only resource your child must express their needs, feelings, and emotions.

It is natural that as a father, you find it annoying, uncomfortable, and sometimes, also frustrating. But you must understand that your child still cannot express in words those emotions and feelings that exceed him. That is, it does not control or manage and, therefore, even less know how to communicate it. Keep calm and arm yourself with endless doses of patience is an indispensable condition to overcome this circumstance. Be willing to talk and explain the number of times that you need the reasons why "no means no."

It is not about handling the situation with authoritarianism, but neither confusing the latter with authority. So, yes, keep a firm and unwavering posture. Of course, also, open to dialogue, communicating with a soft, relaxed, and sincere tone of voice.

Thus, the first thing you should propose is to know the reasons why your child is so angry or upset. The second step is to provide explanations, consequences, and if that is not enough, also propose alternatives. Now, what do you have to tell your son to stop kicking?

Closing phrases to end tantrums.

Your son is going to get everything he has inside, and he won't stop crying and screaming until he gets what he wants. It is not for less since the world has arrived; we have naturally left everything you need at your feet. He knows it, that's why a "no" for him can be something so horrible. The situation will get complicated when you start experiencing things that you don't know how to control or manifest.

But neglect, because, once you have completed the previous steps with temperance, you must play the last card: the closing phrases. Many times, it happens that children end up winning us out of fatigue. Or even getting the worst of us. Many other times, this typical and normal situation leads to an endless sterile struggle for mothers and children.

The idea is that this dialogue can be terminated through a series of sentences.

Of course, they are uttered with total firmness. It's about putting the golden hook when your child doesn't want to understand or plan to continue a meaningless negotiation: nothing but the establishment of an endpoint to any discussion.

The four final phrases of salvation

«I already answered you.» The child may, after all the explanations, consequences, and alternatives provided, try to achieve his goal anyway. One of its methods may be the police-style interrogation that, as you will see, will never end. He will ask, again and again, the same thing that you have already answered many times. The solution is to stop this endless string: answer with an "I already responded" to each reiteration.

"This is no longer in the discussion." When you want to end tantrums that originate from something that you should not allow your child for security reasons, you must be blunt. After the previous steps, if the child insists, close the talk with a «we will not discuss this anymore.» You may seem harsh, but your well-being must be placed above all things.

"This conversation is over." Another right way to close these extensive conversations. Especially when the child returns to the conversation again after hundreds of explanations, if you do not understand the consequences or respond to the alternatives, it is time to end the talk. After finishing this phrase in a firm tone, changing the subject, or looking for another activity will be vital to ending the tantrums.

"The decision is made. If you mention it again, there will be consequences." If your child is very insistent despite having put all your efforts, this is a good option. If you appeal to this strategy, you should be able to comply with it. If, after this phrase, your son still maintains his challenging attitude, it is good to see that you fulfill what you say: «I told you there would be consequences, go to your room and get to do your homework.»

The tantrum stage is good and bad for the child who does not pass it because that means that he has no ideas of his own or that they have crushed him so much that he has stopped defending them.

-Rose Jové-

CHAPTER NINETEEN

Sleep According to Childhood Specialists.

In the Lòczy pedagogy, it is not uncommon to see children sleeping outside, regardless of the temperatures. When creating his structure, Emmi Pikler fitted out two identical living spaces for the child: an outdoor space and an interior space.

In these spaces, the layout of the beds, toys, and all the furniture is the same. The outdoor space is used as much as possible and in all weathers. Indeed, blinds protect children from the cold.

During the winter period, this place is mainly used for napping from the age of one month. Outdoor naps take place at a temperature of minus 10 ° C. Also, Emmi Pikler has established that children, from an early age, are not systematically put back to bed after eating, for example.

Once the child is awake, the child can get up if he can. Otherwise, the adult will pick him up to get him out of bed. The desire to get out of bed is not prohibited. However, the only restriction for children in the structure is to respect the sleep of their peers by being silent and playing calmly. If the young seem tired, they go back to their bed.

According to Maria Montessori (1977), the child should be able to go to bed and wake up when he wishes. For that, it would be necessary to arrange a place by installing a mattress on the floor. This functioning allows the child to be autonomous and to learn to identify and respond to his needs.

Indeed, for this teacher, cribs are objects created for the well-being of the adult. Its purpose is to change the vision that adults have of children. The latter is considered an " Object," which must obey, and which is dependent on the adult. It is, therefore, essential that the adult understands the needs of the child and provides a suitable place for the child to sleep. Thus, the child becomes an actor in his choices.

Huber Montagner, who is a specialist in the development, behavior, and rhythms of children, studied these as well as space in children.

In a book by Michel Margot (1984), which summarizes the conferences which took place for school teachers, we can read that sleep in children takes an essential place for their development and that it needs to be respected and protected. In children, a study shows that the beginning of the afternoon is a period when the ability to concentrate is weaker than the rest of the day.

It is, therefore, important that the child can take a nap to recover when he shows signs of fatigue. Montagner suggests measures that could be taken into consideration by schools, like the introduction of a nap in the early afternoon. For him, parents and all the social workers who gravitate around the child should also be made aware of the fact that sleep is vital for the child's recovery and proper development.

In her book "Living in a crèche, remedying mild violence," Christine Schuhl (2006) names inadequate attitudes which she defines as mild violence, for example, forcing a child to sleep or, on the contrary, not sleeping a child when '' he shows signs of fatigue. We find it essential to list the actions to avoid, according to Ms. Schuhl because these are practices that are not necessarily aware and deemed inappropriate:

- Quickly wake a sleeping child in "do does not wake up" stages

- Chat aloud in the nap rooms while the children are asleep

- Leave the children in bed when they are awake to wait for everyone children to be awake

- Put the sheet on the child's face to help him fall asleep

- Systematically isolate a child from the dormitory Shake a crying child

- Do not take the time to be with the child when he wakes up

In her book, Realizing a Childcare Project (2005), Christine Schuhl recalls that the educational project is compulsory in France. This also applies to Switzerland. It also explains what information, which is highly recommended, should be included in the latter. Among these points, we can find respect for sleep. She develops that it is necessary to accept that the needs of each child are different. Therefore it is essential to individualize the management while taking into account the rhythm of each. At this point also appear the educational postures towards the parents as well as towards the children. She explains that the purpose of an educational project is to make sense of what the instructional team is doing. Thanks to this document, the team has the same bases and can thus be in cohesion.

Sleep in different cultures.

Currently, we live in a multicultural Switzerland made up of different nationalities. In fact, according to the "Valaisan health observatory," Switzerland had 25% of foreigners in 2016. In Valais, 23% of the population is foreign (Valaisan Health Observatory, 2017, population structure, Valais- Swiss).

From the figures above, we can see that there are many different cultures in Switzerland. This mixture appears in the reception structures and can influence the care of the child. Therefore we find it essential to bring examples of cultural practices and to make a link with the difficulties that these differences can cause in educational circles. This point can also provide information on unknown practices that could be taken as courses of action during an issue. Knowing about different exercises can help relativize and perceive specific values in another way.

In our current society, the nap is regulated and limited. We operate in an environment where time is short and where it must be profitable. Certain traditional societies or other cultures do not have the same relation to the nap as we do. However, it can be agreed that napping is essential for everyone. Here are some examples of cultural habits related to napping.

In the Nordic countries, Norway, Finland, or Sweden, napping is done outside. Whatever the season, children can enjoy the long sunny days of summer and the few rays of the sun during the polar winter nights. It has also been proven that the outdoor nap lasts longer than the indoor rest. Parents in Russia expose children to light and outdoor air for a nap. If the little ones sleep inside, it is not uncommon to do so with the windows open.

In China, the nap is "sacred." It is not uncommon for Chinese people to take naps, whether at school or even at work.

A child in Mali sleeps almost 80% of his time on the back of an adult. It is impossible to count the number of naps as well as the duration thereof. However, he will have the same sleep time as a child from our countries. A baby thus sleeps according to its rhythm and the swing of the one who carries it.

In New Caledonia, napping is also practiced by young and old. This is usually done on braided mats, facing the sea and under the coconut trees. Children thus acquire this habit at a very young age.

Indonesian children take longer naps than ours. They are generally performed in a group, or amid their loved ones. Rarely, the child sleeps alone. Sharing a bed with your child is one of the customs.

During one of the nursery interviews, the director explained an anecdote to us. She told us about an event that happened in the structure with a child of African origin whose mother had revealed that she rocked her baby to put him to sleep. So, the instructional staff also practiced this ritual, but it did not work. Until the day the mom came over and showed them how she was doing. Indeed, the difference was evident because it was not the same rocking. That of the mother was very strong, and the director said even to have had the impression that the child was going to fall from the arms. In our culture, we might think that the baby is shaken. We found it interesting that the director also mentioned the fact that all cultures combined have habits that could be found in each of them. She also illustrated this by the example of a Swiss mother who carried her child in a sling to fall asleep.

For the nursery interviewees, the director mentioned that several cultures coexisted in the structure and that she was sometimes confronted with this. Some parents rock their children; others let them fall asleep wherever they want, give them a bottle of milk to fall asleep, etc. However, she tries not to reproduce the rituals of falling asleep at the nursery and tries to make the child fall asleep alone. If it is not the case, then it imitates the gestures of the house. The educator explains to the parents that they are in Switzerland and the community and that the children will have to integrate the rituals of the crèche.

During the interviews, new habits of falling asleep in the child were mentioned. Indeed, on several occasions, the educators, as well as the directors, explained that there are more and more parents who give a bottle of milk to put the child to sleep or who make screens available. These quickly take the place of the ritual of falling asleep. These are not possible in reception structures. Also, according to Dr. Vecchierini, from six months, the baby no longer needs to be fed at night. As for the screens, they propagate a blue light, which has the same effect as daylight. The latter prevents the secretion of melatonin, which favors falling asleep.

CHAPTER TWENTY

The Schematic Sleep Cycles.

Between zero and two months, the infant has a fifty-minute cycle that includes two phases: restless sleep and calm sleep. These stages will repeat for three hours, and it is from about nine weeks that the baby takes a rhythm. The total sleep time is approximately sixteen to twenty hours.

Falling asleep: We can identify it when the baby is not moving apart from a few startles. His face shows very few emotions, as well as specific sucking movements. This phase lasts about twenty minutes.

Restless sleep: This phase of sleep corresponds to REM sleep in adults. During this period, the baby has more and more visible eye movements, the face becomes animated, and the breathing becomes irregular as if the child was going to wake up. This phase is visible when the baby begins to move his fingers, his toes, to stretch and to flex his arms and legs.

His face now expresses the six emotions with facial expressions: surprise, disgust, fear, anger, sadness, and joy with the "smile in heaven." The latter is used to express the moods between living things.

All these expressions already appear in utero; they have been studied and seen through ultrasounds. Sleeping allows the infant to practice expressing them because they are learned and internalized during the first months of life.

As soon as an emotion is made aware and used in a waking state, it will no longer need to be exercised and will disappear during sleep. During this stage, the baby's sleep is restless, and it represents between 50% and 60% of the sleep time until the age of six months. This phase is essential in the baby because he experiences the sensations of the waking state.

Quiet sleep: The sleep phase corresponds to the slow rest in the adult. The baby is practically immobile, and his breathing is calm. There is no eye movement, and his eyes are closed.

Between two cycles: Currently, sleep becomes light. This phase represents the end of a sleep cycle. At this point, the child can either start a new sleep cycle or wake up. When the child resumes a sleep cycle, he can sometimes wake up, have a moment of small awakening during which he will emit short crying, for example.

When the infant wakes up at the end of its sleep cycle, it may find itself in a calm awakening or restless awakening. Sometimes the baby is peaceful and observes his environment, so it represents gentle awakening. Otherwise, he cries and pays little attention to his environment; this represents restless awakening. If the child always wakes up in this way, it is because he has not slept enough during the day.

Between two and six to nine months, the baby's sleep cycle gets longer. The latter's sleep train is made up of three phases: REM sleep, slow sleep, and slow/deep sleep. This cycle lasts seventy minutes. At this period of his life, the baby finally manages to differentiate between day and night.

This acquisition allows him to have a more extended awakening moment during the day. He can also sleep longer at night, thanks to his stomach's capacity to hold more food and thus last longer until the next meal. At around three months, the baby can sleep for seven to eight hours continuously.

The sleep phases are, therefore: REM sleep, which corresponds to restless sleep in infants, slow sleep, which corresponds to calm rest in infants, and we end up with slow/deep sleep. C is from six months that can be observed in sleep characteristics that refer to the sleep of adults. At this time of life, the recommended number of hours of sleep is sixteen hours.

Slow / deep sleep: This sleep phase is the most restorative. When a child is in it, it is usually tough to wake it up. Currently, the muscles are all relaxed; the brain and the whole organism are at rest. This phase is essential for recovery and is, therefore, very important.

Between two and six months, the baby thinks of forming a single person with his mother. After this stage, the child understands that he is a being in his own right. C 'is the beginning of the construction of the "me," especially studied by Freud. The baby will then be afraid of losing his mother and will need to find a substitute for this attachment figure. Generally, parents offer replacement items, but the child often makes the final choice. This stable object, generally handy and sometimes impregnated with the smell of its mother and called "transitional object" by Winnicott or, more commonly, "comforter."

The latter therefore allows the baby to feel secure even when his attachment figure is absent and to become independent at different times of the day. Being stable and permanent, the object can be beneficial during falling asleep and the awakenings that arise during sleep. The child will not need to call the adult when he feels insecure or in distress during the day. This transitional object is very often used during the nap moment so that the child can feel safe during the time of falling asleep.

According to Researchers, it is not for the professionals of childhood to decide if the child should or should not have these objects called transitional. This decision rests with the parents and the child. Therefore she recommends having bins in the living room that are accessible to children and in which the cuddly toys, coats, and the child's personal belongings are located. However, in the two structures that I interviewed, the babies ' personal belongings were not accessible to them. The cuddly toys and coats are generally given during moments of the nap or when the child expresses by crying during the day. Indeed, here, it is the adult who decides to give these transitional objects.

Between nine and eighteen months, the naps of the day decrease. Up to twelve months, the child takes three naps: in the morning, at the beginning of the afternoon, and the end of the afternoon. From this age, the afternoon nap disappears. The phases present in the sleep cycle are the same as in the age group of two to nine months. However, the order of the phases changes, and they are ordered as follows: slow sleep, deep, slow sleep, and REM sleep. However, the duration of the cycle remains the same, seventy minutes. The total sleep duration, from nine months, is approximately fifteen hours.

CHAPTER TWENTY-ONE

Toddler Sleep Disorders - How to Detect a Problem and Get the Right Help.

During each stage of life, different conditions can occur, which affect children differently. Each elderly child may react to these conditions separately. Toddler sleep disorders are very similar in any other developmental stage to the disorders. Treatments differ because a baby is still developing, and their body is going through constant changes. The easiest way to avoid a sleep disorder and a sleep clinic's evaluation is to stop a disorder from ever occurring. Training your child to sleep alone and fall asleep on their own makes a big difference about whether your child is suffering from one of these conditions or not. Establishing a good sleep schedule is one of the best things you can do to ensure good sleep and healthy growth for your children.

Some simple instructions will help you work with your child and get in a good routine. Connection at night should be prohibited. Consistent holding, singing, and petting will lead to wanting your child to fall asleep and required those acts. This dependence will prevent them from falling asleep by themselves when bedtime arrives. Every day, unexciting rituals should be used just before bedtime. Such things can be stuff like meditation, story time, or a bath. They have to be done every night, so your child feels safe and comfortable.

Do not require coffee beverages. Regular routines and bedtime help the body adapt and make it more comfortable to sleep and wake. Their bed should be used to relax and not to allow time to play. When an infant spends an awake amount of time in bed, it becomes less likely to sleep there.

It is not possible to avoid all infantile sleep disorders. There are parasomnias, apnea, and nightmares all popular. Some parasomnias overcome themselves like night terrors and sleepwalking. When they seriously interrupt your child's sleep, it is highly recommended that you discuss options for reducing incidents or mitigating the impact with your doctor. Apnea and other conditions of sleep may require a sleep clinic evaluation and specific treatments to make your child's rest more relaxed and more welcoming. If you are worried that your child may have a sleep disorder, control their sleep for a couple of nights to see if there are any evident signs.

Further testing is sometimes necessary to determine the cause of the sleep disturbances. Often a pediatrician will test for other medical conditions that could contribute to the problem. We can suggest improvements that can be tried to help at home. A referral to a specialist can be provided for more severe issues. Such specialists are familiar with all the disorders which affect children and infants in general.

They have access to specific facilities that facilitate the testing and diagnosis. Through equipment and the naked eye, your child can be tracked as they sleep in a comfortable environment. The outcomes of these assessments are used to assess if there is a condition, its extent, and what treatment options are available. With a few simple tests, your child can sleep well again, and have all they need to lead a healthier life.

Tips For Solving Toddler Sleep Disorders.

Young children need several hours of sleep each day, and it is your responsibility to make sure they get it. Some children are advised to have a total of twelve hours of rest during the night, and at least one but ideally not less than two hours of rest during the daytime. If your child simply doesn't want to stop long enough to go to bed, this becomes a problem. These 6 tips will help your baby sleep better and easier.

Build a nap and bedtime routine and make your child abide by it. Children who are placed in bed and nap at the same time each day rest well and go down more quickly than children who are allowed to fall asleep when they become too tired to stay awake any longer. Once a child gets used to a routine, they are exhausted when the usual time comes.

Whenever you put your baby to sleep, make your room as quiet and comfortable as possible. Switch off or lower lights, which are usually turned on when playing. Play calming music as background noise to help them calm down and take away any and all toys except protective things such as special blankets or stuffed animals. Try recreating the calming atmosphere whenever you want to lay down your boy.

Children depend on routines, although they do not learn. Have individual acts that you do if your child lays down and do them regularly. Make sure such acts can go down when your child is lying in his or her own bed. You want to avoid behaviors such as rocking or laying down with them, as you might not always be able to do so. Storytime is expected to come at the end of this cycle while they're still tucked in bed.

Young children should never watch a lot of television, and that is particularly important before bedtime. Loud TV shows and cartoons can increase their hyperactivity and over-stimulation. It made calming down and relaxed enough to get some proper rest more difficult for them.

Make sure your child doesn't need anything to make it more difficult for them to rest. Giving them plenty to eat and drink before going to bed is time for them, so they don't try to sleep on empty stomachs. Changing diapers at this time would be a good idea if they're not already toilet trained.

Screaming and yelling about making your child rest can often have the opposite effect. It only helps to annoy and make the child confused. You don't always understand why you scream and what you did wrong. When talking to them, it is best to remain calm, as this will help keep them quiet.

CHAPTER TWENTY-TWO

How to Help Your Child through Night Terrors.

Toddler Night Terrors is common in children. Beginning at age three, as your child grows older, her imagination begins to become more active. There comes to fear, along with an active imagination. A Toddler can have a hard time distinguishing between imagination and reality. As a society, we train children to be afraid of the dark through movies and TV shows. It's out of the dark, "that the terrifying evil monsters show." So, it's no wonder that children start hearing and seeing monsters and ghosts everywhere, alone in their beds at night. Dr. Richard Sherman, a Los Angeles clinical psychologist, says, "Monster fear is real, it's a very common problem among children aged 3 to 6."

Night terrors for the parent too can be very exhausting. If your child wakes up begging to reach your bedroom, it leads to long nights. Simply give in when you're tired and let your child hop with you into your bed. Try not to make a habit of that, though, or he will never overcome his fear.

Here are some ideas that could work with your child to help him develop Healthy Sleep Habits and therefore be a more comfortable Child at Night.

- The most important thing to do is to be compassionate and helpful. I know how hard it can be for your boy, who's just had a nightmare, to be awakened at 2 am, exhausted and restless.

Getting cranky is simple, but note that for your child, this is a legitimate fear, so be understanding. Don't yell at him; help him conquer his terror.

- Hours before going to bed, make sure that the positive messages surround your children. Consider stopping TV 2 hours before going to bed, even Transformers or Harry Potter will help you work your imagination up. A program for an innocent child, named Little Bear, had an episode in Halloween where the Little Bear saw a goblin. For you, this may seem harmless enough, but he is not your boy.

- Try to develop a sedentary routine before bedtime. Have your child take a bath or read the story of a kind child that will fill him with happy pictures.

- During the night, have a nightlight on to help. You could even find night lights inspired by Disney's favorite character for your children.

- Leave the door open, and if your room is close to your child's, let him hear your voice so he knows you're not far away while he can't see you.

- Play some soft music in his house or have handy tapes of stories. Let him focus on the story or music and not on his imagination.

- It's okay to have the child sleep with you on occasions until this stage is over. What matters is that you're ok with it. If it upsets your rest to the extent that the next day you'll be anxious and cranky, then try another approach.

- Make sure you talk to your child about his anxieties. Don't play down on them. To her, they are real. If your child tells you that there is a demon in the closet, don't say that you get rid of that. He would presume that you also believe in monsters, and she will feel that they really do exist.

- Practice visualization strategies with your children. Help her train her mind when her nocturnal fear begins to think of something optimistic or funny.

- Try repeating several times, "you are safe" when your child is crying out.

- It's okay to stay by her side sometimes until she falls asleep. But don't repeat it often, or your child will rely on you being next to her to fall asleep.

- As an alternative to number 11, check-in regularly on your children, spreading check-in times at any time. The first check-in, for example, will be in 5 minutes, second in 10 minutes, third in 15 minutes, etc. when the baby sleeps. Depending on the level of fear of your child, you may start the first check-in the next night in 10 min.

If your child's fears have crossed the line, being inconsolable, it may be anxiety or a phobia. Or a symptom of an underlying emotional disorder owing to a stressful event or a sudden change in the life of your child. Consult with your child's medical professional whenever in doubt.

CHAPTER TWENTY-THREE

Motor Development Milestones and Baby's Sleep 4 - 12 Months.

Here is a list of milestones in motor growth-how they can affect sleep, and what you can do to help your baby get back on track. A recent study reported a link between the emergence of night waking and motor development milestones-babies were found to have a tougher time settling to sleep and would start waking more often at night, two weeks before taking their first steps. It's also important to remember that babies still wake up at night and like to practice their newly found skills because it's so much more fun than going to sleep-in fact, they want to whine a little or call you to join them for their late-night rendezvous.

- **4 - 6 months**

Rolling back to front from their back but not being able to move around.

Once a baby starts rolling, the above example will have you on the back a few times in the night to help the baby rollback. If you haven't seen them rolling backward from their tummy, then they probably haven't mastered the ability yet - so you might need to help first. Nonetheless, once you've seen them do it - you should refrain from getting too involved; otherwise, they'll call on you to come and do it every time. Once an infant can roll over the muscles of the neck, it becomes smoother, and the risk of SIDS diminishes. Many parents worry about their baby and this tragic phenomenon, but there's no need to worry about it, your baby usually develops and builds even more strength for their next incredible step.

- **6- 9 month**

Sitting - Crawling & Standing

Sitting - Once a baby has grown into their head, they are no longer so heavy, and finally, they can sit down. You may find that once you're in bed, you can go from being on your back to rolling to pushing up quickly and get up flat in 5 seconds. This can be especially challenging for co-sleeping parents once there is little one awake and sat up, they think it's super fun to poke your eye and touch your nose while simultaneously practicing the odd vowel or delightful squeal. You should tackle this by putting them back down and saying a keyword or "shhh" in a calm and collective manner, limiting eye contact and doing nothing to get them excited about thinking it's morning time. Sometimes, they can sit back up but lay them back down again.

Crawling-This is the one you've been waiting for for-starting to crawl your little sugar plum, and then, when it happens, you realize you've had so much more control when they're just sitting. If your baby crawls on all fours, using their hands, with butt in the air and their legs like they're walking, or sitting on their bum and scooting around in reverse, this is another little wrench in the sleep works for you!

Babies just love to practice this kind of nighttime stuff when they wake up during their light sleep phase. You put them to bed in one place, and they're squashed in the corner the next time you see them, with a blanket wrapped around their limbs looking somewhat like a pretzel.

Crawling can also create anxiety about separation as your little one starts to understand that they are not an object to you but a separate entity of their own. This form of stress has a distinctive cry that parents sometimes characterize as more of a scream or hysteria and can cause quite a bit of regression of sleep.

- **9 - 12 months plus**

Walking, another night blow for you, during these milestones, your little one won't stop, because they want to discover all the possible avenues, yes, they'll wake up at night and practice scaling the cradle, walking from top to bottom, be vigilant and refrain If you have something troublesome in the crib that could be a danger and if you need to put on a crib bumper or protection.

Offer plenty of opportunities to explore and use their energy throughout the day for your little one. At this age, they barely stop for breathing. Babies never like being confined to their sleeping positions or squeezed into car seats at this age. While your little one is full of energy that they are just waiting to burn off, they still need a decent amount of sleep, so don't be fooled into thinking that naps are not necessary just because your baby doesn't show signs of slowing. They still need about 11-12 hours of night sleep at this age and 2-3 hours of two naps during the day.

CHAPTER TWENTY-FOUR

Bedtime Pass, a Method That Helps Children Sleep.

The Bedtime pass can be the solution for children to sleep better, do not resist sleeping and sleep in their bed for the estimated time for it. Its effectiveness is proven.

Bedtime can become a stressful affair for the family. Screaming, crying, fear, anguish, and uninterrupted sleep and wake up can become routine when we don't have an effective method to manage this problem. Fortunately, there are some like the Bedtime pass.

Sometimes, we may come to think that it only happens to our family, but calmly, we can all go through these difficulties. The important thing is to find how to act assertively to achieve a peaceful and restful sleep in each of the family members.

Bedtime pass, what is it?

It is ubiquitous that children do not want to go to bed at bedtime. The reasons can be many, let's see some:

- They prefer to stay longer playing.

- They want to spend more time with their family.

- For rebellion.

- They feel fear (to be left unattended, to the darkness, to the nightmares).

There can be many causes; therefore, we must review all those routines that surround the dream. What does the child do when the hours before going to sleep? What do you do if you wake up at night?

A practical method that helps children sleep is the Bedtime pass. It is a viable technique to use in children who have difficulties or rejection at bedtime. In addition, it is supported by different investigations.

The difficulties that are usually addressed in this method are the resistance of going to bed and falling asleep. Also, resist participating in the routine of going to bed, calling from the bed, or leaving the room after going to bed or waking up at night. What happens is that behaviors are reinforced or sustained by the delay in bedtime and maintaining contact with caregivers.

For this, the Bedtime pass can be an appropriate strategy. In fact, it is also advisable, for children who can initiate sleep independently in their own beds or rooms.

How to implement the Bedtime pass?

The Bedtime Pass is a way to teach our little ones to be in their bed and sleep independently, with minimal protests. Let's see what steps to follow according to this model:

- Sit with the child and explain what we are going to do.

- Explain to the child that he has trouble sleeping and that you have an idea of how to help him. For example, you can say: "I know it's hard for you to sleep, so I thought of an idea."

- Explain the strategy to the child as follows. «You and I will make a pass for you to use every night, you will get a night pass» After mom and dad have put you to bed, you can use the pass for a free trip outside the room, it must be for a specific reason, For example, go to the bathroom, hug mom and dad. If you use the pass, you must give it to us (to mom to dad or to the caregiver), and then go back to bed».

- It should be emphasized that there must be a specific brief reason (approximately 5 minutes).

- Explain what happens after the child has already used the pass. For example, "After using the pass, you must go back to bed and stay there for the rest of the night."

- Make the pass with your child (ren)—the more creative, the better. You must allow the child to participate.

- Just before bedtime, you must give your child the pass and remind him of the purpose.

- If your child uses the pass, allow it, take the pass and remind him that after using it, it is time to stay in his room and remain silent.

Now, if your child calls you after using the pass, it would be to ignore this behavior, even if he insists. And, if you leave the room after using the pass, you must guide him back to his room physically, without speaking. Remember to impose these rules with a head, assessing that the level of suffering does not exceed certain limits.

The first night it is essential to remember the rules to your child until they are internalized. Also, don't forget to reward your child for using the pass and staying in his room after that. If you are consistent, the chances of success will increase. Also, make sure other people who take care of your child maintain this routine.

What are the benefits of Bedtime pass?

Since you have seen what this method is about and how to carry it out, we show you the main advantages of using it, let's see:

- The child will quickly learn that it is better to keep the pass since not doing so will not receive attention, as he wishes.

- It reduces discomfort when going to bed.

- It is a plus for sleep hygiene.

- Resistance to sleep can be eliminated.

- Decrease resistance to sleep independently.

- Increase the level of satisfaction.

- It provides parents and children with an element of control.

- It decreases the anguish.

- Assertive emotional management is enhanced.

- Improves the ability to make decisions.

Although there are all these benefits it is appropriate to remind you, that at the beginning of the child insists on maintaining protest behaviors, it can be distressing not to go to him, but with the passage of time when you see the results that anguish should decrease, as well as such behaviors.

How to develop social skills in children.

Developing correct social skills in children will not only help them build more positive relationships or interact much better with others. What we will put at your fingertips is the real core of social and emotional learning, where empathy and assertiveness constitute by themselves two indisputable psychic tendons.

Let us now ask ourselves a simple question: " How do our children really learn?" As multiple studies on social psychology tell us, and even as Albert Bandura himself revealed to us with his experiments, children develop most of their learning through observation, Imitation, and continuous interaction.

Social skills can be somewhat complicated since they are integrated from feelings, beliefs, values and a whole repertoire of strategies with which to ensure that the child survives and progresses in a healthy way in his social and emotional journey.

Of all these processes, of course, we call them "sociability" and form for themselves a decisive foundation in the child's life. Thus, depending on the quality of the same and the experiences, the perceptions, attributions built, and the socio-emotional learning assumed, healthy and productive social skills will be shaped or, conversely, a series of deficiencies that usually be very problematic arrival already pre-adolescence.

On the other hand, something that experts in child psychology tell us very often is that the social reality of today is much more complicated for children than it was at the time for their parents. The media, new technologies, and the constantly changing rules of our society place our little ones in a field that is large and for which they do not have a compass with which to locate.

The ways of relating and even meeting people have changed, social networks or messaging services are more dynamic, offer new opportunities, are faster, lack filters, control mechanisms, and instants, of course, are quite dangerous.

It is positive that the social development of children covers many areas, many areas, and new scenarios. It is vital to make available those tools, enough and necessary so that they can function effectively and healthily in an increasingly intricate social sphere, more extensive, but also valuable, after all. Hence the importance of learning social skills in children.

The development of social skills in children.

One of the most effective strategies for developing social skills in children is to develop a very early "common language." First, we are speaking of an understandable, simple, and efficient type of language that even 2-year-olds can understand.

Recall that this age is a crucial moment in your child's development. Now it's when he starts claiming his new sovereignty, describing his character and being much more open to all that's going on around him.

This social language that will favor the early development of social skills in children is based on the following dimensions:

- Learn to practice active listening. We cannot speak while the other person is saying something; we must respect times. This is something that costs them because their self-control is still minimal. On the other hand, the best way to teach them is by example: if we don't interrupt them, they will learn not to interrupt us.

- The little ones must learn to show gratitude, to know when and how to apologize, and to include a "please" in their demands. Let us teach them, either implicitly or explicitly, the difference between a request and a requirement.

- The appropriate social language also includes different "pearls of wisdom": that of giving us positive reinforcements, knowing how to say "thank you," knowing how to tolerate, knowing how to share, recognizing when others do something right and when it is I who is wrong.

Help them form a positive image of themselves.

Getting our children to learn to value themselves, to love each other and to protect their rights and identity, is to invest in their quality of life and to give wings to their personal potential. However, how to achieve it? Sometimes we are so immersed in favoring in them the curricular competencies and in getting them to be good in mathematics and proficient in English that we completely neglect the most essential: supporting a positive image of themselves.

Keys to promote good self-esteem in children.

Be your best model. Be your best reference and a figure to imitate in everyday life.

- **Spend quality time with your children.** It is not just about being "present," but about your presence being nutritious, flattering, and inspiring.

- **Offer them opportunities.** The little one who feels competent builds a correct self-esteem every day.

- **Avoid labels at all costs, do not compare it with other children or with your siblings or with any other person.** That child is unique, valuable, and capable of doing incredible things for himself.

- **Always value your efforts.** Also, before resorting to mere sanction or negative criticism, teach them what the right way to do things is.

CHAPTER TWENTY-FIVE

Sleep and sleep disorders.

The process of sleep and wakefulness is controlled primarily by a biological clock or natural rhythm, which controls the elimination of sleep and hunger. The child's circadian rhythms (natural 24-hour rhythms) are very different from those of adults. Thus, the newborn spends most of his time (about 18 hours a day) sleeping from birth. The baby wakes up every two or three hours (day and night) to be nourished for about three months. Approximately six months old, a baby will spend several hours a night (five or six) without waking up: it's said he's making the nights. The cycle of this baby consists of peaceful sleep cycles and restless sleep periods (around 50 percent). For adults, active sleep is associated with REM sleep. Throughout the lifetime, this type of sleep decreases to about 20% of the total sleep time.

The infant's sleep activity induces results in the parents or other careers. A child who sleeps well and is happy gives a sense of confidence to parents. On the contrary, in his setting, a child who sleeps little and is restless (crying) is provoking irritability, even exasperation. Some parents (because of the baby's lack of education, stress, or unrealistic expectations) may also shake their baby to try to silence him. This action can cause severe brain damage or even death (shaken baby syndrome) that is permanent.

An infant sleeps an average of 13 hours a day around the age of two (mainly at night, and a little as a nap during the day). This figure varies from country to country based on cultural factors affecting parental ethno-theories (the parents' implicit theories) and associated parenting practices. He spends less time sleeping as the child grows older. Five-year-olds sleep 12 hours during the night on average and don't sleep anymore. Six-year-olds have an average 11-hour sleep requirement; those twelve, a 9-hour sleep.

Rituals of the child's bedtime.

Bedtime may cause anxiety about separation in children who may sometimes want to resist. Parents can help the child make the time more comfortable and less frustrating by creating a bedtime routine or ritual. The approach is advised to be consistent and straightforward, "including a fixed time for bedtime and bedtime routines that are calm and do not go on." Techniques may include reading aloud children's books, the rhymes. The presence of a soft cloth or toy with smooth texture helps children feel more peaceful. Thus, the pediatrician and psychoanalyst Donald Winnicott described objects of attachment as transitional objects, helping the child to better live the separations (a blanket, a soft toy).

Child's sleep disorders.

Children may have difficulty sleeping. The nightmares are quite normal. These usually occur at the end of the night, and the child retains the memory. They're more prevalent in girls than boys. Frequent nightmares that make the anxious child during periods of waking indicate excessive stress.

Night terrors differ from nightmare terrors. The child appears to suddenly wake up in a state of panic from deep sleep (he may scream or stare in front of him) but does not remember a dream. He goes back to sleep and wakes up without even remembering the episode. Night terrors occur more frequently in boys and are more often observed between three and 13 years.

Sleepwalking (the sleepwalking act) and sleep talking (speaking while sleeping) is popular among children as well. Hoban (2004) suggests not waking a child who is sleepwalking or a child who has developed a nightmare of the night so as not to disturb him. Such sleep disturbances usually go away over time.

Bedwetting (urinating while sleeping) is also common in children. Enuresis affects about 10-15% of 5-year-olds and then decreases with age.

- ***Developmental disorders.***

Developmental conditions arise from fetal, perinatal, or early infancy and are typically the result of brain dysfunction. Developmental disorders refer to a category of heterogeneous and chronic disorders that have the characteristic of disrupting developmental skill acquisition or perception.

These developmental skills include fine and gross motor skills, language, personal and social competencies, cognition, and daily living activities. Such domains are neither wholly separate nor mutually exclusive. The most extreme pathologies are usually recognized earlier than the lesser and more common modest types.

Developmental disorders include cerebral palsy, developmental delay, mental disability, primary language disorder or dysphasia, autism spectrum disorder (ASD), attention deficit and hyperactivity disorder (ADHD), learning disabilities, coordination acquisition disorder (TAC), and genetic and chromosomal anomalies.

Because the developmental conditions stem from brain damage, they are persistent and permanent. These are non-progressive, though, which means that the underlying cause is not progressive and that these diseases are not causing death. The developmental nature of development, however, makes the illness symptoms as well as the child's psychological image-problems, needs, attitudes, etc.-change over time.